ATKINS

Atkins Diet Plan 2019

The New Losing Weight With Atkins Diet For A Beginner's Guide and Step by step Simpler Way to Lose Weight.

Katherine Hannah

Copyright © 2019 by Katherine Hannah

All rights reserved.

No part of this book may be reproduced in any form or by any electronic or mechanical means, including information storage and retrieval systems, without written permission from the author, except for the use of brief quotations in a book review.

TABLE OF CONTENTS

WHAT TYPES OF MEALS SHOULD YOU EAT ON ATKINS DIET? 7

ATKINS DIET PLAN: 8

START WITH THE ATKINS DIET 13

YOU CAN FOLLOW THESE RECIPES FOR GOOD DIET!..16

STUFFED CHICKEN WITH ASPARAGUS & BACON...16

BASIL STUFFED CHICKEN BREASTS..18

5 MINUTE LOW CARB CHICKEN NUGGETS 20

SAUSAGE KALE SOUP WITH MUSHROOM..21

BUNLESS BURGER 22

WHITE LASAGNA STUFFED PEPPERS 24

CREAMY BASIL BAKED SAUSAGE 26

LOW CARB PORK MEDALLIONS 28

EASY MOZZARELLA & PESTO CHICKEN CASSEROLE 30

EASY TACO CASSEROLE RECIPE..32

PARMESAN CHICKEN TENDERS...34

BROCCOLI & CHEDDAR KETO BREAD RECIPE 36

BACON WRAPPED CHICKEN TENDERS WITH RANCH DIP..................................37

FARMHOUSE BEANS & SAUSAGE 39

CHICKEN AL FORNO & VODKA SAUCE WITH TWO CHEESES 41

STUFFED PORK CHOPS – 5 INGREDIENTS 42

SUPER EASY SPICY BAKED CHICKEN 44

LEMON PARMESAN BROCCOLI SOUP 46

MEAT-LOVER PIZZA CUPS 48

FRESH TOMATO BASIL SOUP 50

RANCH YOGURT MARINADE FOR GRILLED CHICKEN 52

5 MINUTE 5 INGREDIENT CHEESY BACON CHICKEN 53

BAKED PESTO CHICKEN 54

PIZZA CHICKEN CASSEROLE 56

KETO CAULIFLOWER AU GRATIN 57

BOOSTED KETO COFFEE 59

SUGAR FREE LOW CARB DRIED CRANBERRIES 60

KETO HOLLANDAISE 61

KETO SAUSAGE BALLS 63

PORK BELLY WEDGE SALAD 64

PICKLED RED ONIONS 65

DAIRY FREE KETO RANCH DRESSING 67

CREAMY CHIVE BLUE CHEESE DRESSING 69

BLACK BEAUTY – LOW CARB VODKA DRINK 70

LOW CARB TORTILLA PORK RIND WRAPS 72

KETO HONEY MUSTARD CHICKEN 74

EVERYTHING BUT THE BAGEL SEASONING 76

KETO DAIRY FREE SHAMROCK SHAKE 77

KETO HONEY MUSTARD DRESSING 78

CRISPY BAKED GARLIC PARMESAN WINGS 79

LOW CARB STRAWBERRY MARGARITA GUMMY 81

HERBED CHICKEN AND MUSHROOMS 83

PUMPKIN SPICE ROASTED PECANS 85

LOW CARB KETO BANANA NUT PROTEIN PANCAKES 86

CHOCOLATE PEANUT BUTTER NO BAKE COOKIES 88

LOW CARB KETO NUT FREE PIZZA CRUST 90

LOW CARB WHOLE30 ALMOND COCONUT MILK CREAMER	92
PALEO 2 MINUTE AVOCADO OIL MAYO	94
KETO SAUSAGE AND EGG BREAKFAST SANDWICH	96
HOT CRAB AND ARTICHOKE DIP	97
ROASTED RED PEPPER GARLIC AIOLI	99
LOW CARB TURKEY CLUB PINWHEELS	100
LOW CARB CAULIFLOWER RICE MUSHROOM RISOTTO	102
KETO CHILI DOG POT PIE CASSEROLE	104
LOW CARB CROCK POT PIZZA CASSEROLE	106
LOW CARB TACO CASSEROLE	108
EASY LOW CARB BREAKFAST CASSEROLE	110
CHEESY CHICKEN AND BROCCOLI CASSEROLE	112
SPINACH AND MUSHROOM BREAKFAST CASSEROLE	114
ALFREDO SAUCE RECIPE	116
ALMOND & COCONUT FLOUR MUFFIN IN A MUG	117
CAPRESE SNACK	119
ORIENTAL RED CABBAGE SALAD	120
SALAD IN A JAR	122
COLESLAW	124
ASPARAGUS AND LEEK SOUP	126
ASIAN LOBSTER SALAD	128
SIAN-STYLE COLESLAW	130
2 INGREDIENT LOW CARB CREPES	132

ATKINS DIET PLAN 2019

WHAT TYPES OF MEALS SHOULD YOU EAT ON ATKINS DIET?

Protein- and fat-rich meals are in; carbs are out. In the primary weeks, you will ceremonial dinner nearly solely on carb-loose fares like meat, fish, shellfish, hen, and eggs, even though low-carb greens are authorized. As you move via the stages, you'll progressively reacquaint yourself with extra carbs – a slice of bread, perhaps, a dash of dairy, a handful of nuts, a few fruit or legumes.

The shape those ingredients take is as much as you. You've got many delicacies alternatives – from Mexican to Italian to Asian – at your disposal, in addition to the steerage of a handful of Atkins-recommended cooks. And for folks who assume a stove just takes up precious space, Atkins sells a line of low-carb bars and shakes.

ATKINS DIET PLAN:

The Atkins diet is a popular diet plan that is based on eating low carbohydrates. How much you lose differs per person, but in general, you lose weight quickly if you eat little carbohydrates. There are a few phases within the Atkins diet, the initial phase of which is usually the most difficult. This initial phase can have several typical side effects because you eat very few carbohydrates. These include headache, moodiness, bad breath, fatigue, bowel changes, and mental fatigue. Although the first stage of the Atkins diet can be difficult, it is certainly worth it in the long run.

- Drink coffee and tea. A typical side effect of following a low-carbohydrate diet such as the Atkins diet is that the body system is in a state of ketosis. That means that your body will get energy from ketones instead of glucose (a carbohydrate), as it normally does. Headache is one of the consequences that is the most common.

An easy and natural way to get rid of the headache is to drink something with caffeine in it. Research has shown that a little caffeine can relieve the headache.

Headache often occurs when the blood vessels in the brain expand, causing them to press against the skull. Caffeine causes the vessels to contract again so that they become thinner, reducing the pain.

Caffeine works quickly, and you usually notice relief within 30 minutes. The effect lasts for three to five hours.

Both coffee and tea are sources of caffeine, but coffee contains more caffeine. A 240 ml cup of coffee contains between 80 and 200 mg of caffeine. Drink one or two cups to relieve the headache.

Although you also find caffeine in soft drinks, sports drinks, and energy drinks, these drinks are not on the list of approved drinks within the Atkins diet.

- Try self-care products. In addition to headaches, ketosis, and a low-carbohydrate diet can also make you feel nauseous and change bowel movements. By taking self-care products, you can reduce these side effects.

If a cup of hot coffee does not help against the headache, you can take a painkiller. They are safe for most healthy people to use and provide relief from pain. Also, you can opt for a painkiller with caffeine, so that the medicine works faster and more effectively.

If you notice that you are clogged or have diarrhea, you can also take a self-care remedy to alleviate these side effects. Take a mild laxative or a fiber supplement if you cannot go to the toilet. If you are hidden too long, it will get worse, and you will need more aggressive treatment, such as an enema.

Nausea is a different side effect that can make the first days or weeks of the Atkins diet more difficult. Drink ginger tea or ginger ale, but avoid dairy products, because that can make you sicker. You can also take a self-care remedy for nausea.

- Beat peppermints and sugar-free chewing gum. Another temporary side effect of the Atkins diet is bad breath. Again, this is often due to ketosis, but you can easily remedy it.

A good way to avoid bad breath is to brush your teeth regularly. Consider bringing a travel toothbrush and a small tube of toothpaste. Brush more often than usual and also thoroughly brush the back of your tongue.

There are also mouthwashes that contain antibacterial components that can help fight bad breath.

In addition to a strict oral care regime, you can suck on mints or chew sugar-free chewing gum. Make sure you pay good attention to whether the amount of sugars fits within your diet.

- Don't do too much. It is normal for you to be a little tired or drowsy the first few days or weeks of the Atkins diet. Limit your physical exercise until these side effects are over.

Because the Atkins diet restricts you a bit, especially about the number of carbohydrates, you don't have to physically exhaust yourself.

It is recommended to do moderate to intensive cardio training for 150 minutes every week, as well as strength training for one to two days a week. This can be a bit too much at the start of your diet. Instead of doing moderate to intensive cardio training, you can try to do the same amount of not too intensive cardio. Activities such as walking or quiet cycling may be easier and more fun if you stick to a strict diet.

Exercise can also provide a positive mentality if your diet is difficult to sustain.

- Go to bed earlier. It is not surprising that you are a little tired or even grumpy during the first days of the Atkins diet. Make sure you sleep enough to counteract these effects.

You need seven to nine hours of sleep every night. If you don't touch it now, you will find that you get really tired and drowsy if you eat little carbohydrates.

Try to go to bed a little quicker each day during the first phase of the Atkins diet. Stay a little longer if you can.

- Set up a support group. It can be useful to have a support group with every diet so that you can encourage each other and keep up better.

Many studies show that people who are supported by friends or family maintain a diet better and lose more weight than people without a support group.

Tell your friends or family that you are going to follow the Atkins diet and say how much you want to lose weight. Ask if they want to support you and if they might want to join you.

Also, you will find all sorts of options for seeking support on the Atkins diet website. Take a look at their website for more information.

- Seek support. There will be challenges with every diet. If you have a group of people that you support, you will get more motivation and encouragement to stick to your new diet.

Ask friends, families, and colleagues to support you. Tell them about your new diet and your long-term goals. Maybe they even want to participate.

A support group can also assist you with the mental difficulties of following a diet. It can be a challenge to maintain a strict diet such as the Atkins diet day in, day out.

Research has revealed that people who have a support group maintain a diet longer, stick to it better, and lose more weight than people who don't.

- Start a diary. Keeping a diary about your new diet and long-term goals can be a good way to deal with the difficulties associated with following such a diet. Sometimes writing in a diary alone is enough to keep you on the right track.

Use a pen and notebook or an online app to start a diary. You don't have to write every day, but it helps to put your thoughts on paper.

You can also use your diary to keep track of your progress.

START WITH THE ATKINS DIET

- View which foods and recipes are allowed. When you start a new diet, you first have to understand what it means, and what you can and cannot eat. Then the transition to the diet is a lot easier.

The Atkins diet is a very particular type of low-carbohydrate diet. It is divided into four phases with a separate list of foods and portion sizes that are allowed within each phase.

In phase 1 you are allowed to eat full-fat cheese, fats, and oil, fish and shellfish, poultry, eggs, meat, herbs, vegetables that do not contain starch and green leafy vegetables (the so-called basic vegetables).

Stock up on these foods so that you have everything that is permitted within reach to prepare meals and snacks.

- Eat every two to three hours. Eating every few hours will prevent you from getting hungry, but it is especially advisable during the first phase of the Atkins diet.

With this diet, it is recommended to eat three meals plus two snacks a day or to eat five to six small meals a day. Make sure you never wait longer than three hours to eat.

If you sit between meals or snacks for more than three hours, you get too hungry and are more likely to eat something that is not allowed because you are starving.

Always take a meal or snack with you when you go out. Then you avoid eating something that is not on the allowed list when you get hungry.

- Eat the right amount of carbohydrates. You will notice that during each phase of the Atkins diet, a very specific amount of carbohydrates per day is recommended. It is important to follow this guideline very carefully.

During the first phase of the diet, you are allowed 20 grams of carbohydrates per day. It is expedient not to exceed that amount, but also to ensure that you eat at least 18 grams of carbohydrates.

If you eat less than 18 grams of carbohydrates, you do not lose weight earlier, but you probably do not eat enough basic vegetables.

Spread the 20 grams of carbohydrates throughout the day. This makes you feel more even throughout the day. If you take all 20 grams of carbohydrates for breakfast, you will experience more side effects in the afternoon.

- Drink enough. With the Atkins diet, as with most other diets, it is recommended to drink a lot.

Water is essential for your overall health, even if you are not on a diet. Also, drinking enough, as previously mentioned, can prevent nausea and blockage.

The Atkins diet suggests drinking at least eight large glasses of water a day. General guidelines even suggest that you should drink 13 glasses of water a day. This depends on your age, gender, and level of activity.

You should not be thirsty all day, and your urine should be clear at the end of the day if you have drunk enough.

- Consider taking supplements. The Atkins diet recommends that you maintain Phase 1 for at least two weeks or until you are 5 - 7 pounds away from your goal weight. If you want to lose a lot of weight, you may have to take dietary supplements.

The initial stage of the Atkins diet does extremely limited and removes various food groups (such as fruit, starchy vegetables, and grains) from your diet. If you plan to maintain this phase for a longer period, it is a good idea to take dietary supplements to prevent you from getting a shortage of certain nutrients.

A multivitamin is a good "backup." Take one a day to ensure that you get all the necessary nutrients every day.

You can also consider taking 500-1000 mg of calcium per day because you do not eat dairy.

Tips

Don't neglect to get 12 to 15 grams of carbohydrates from your basic vegetables per day. The fibers in these vegetables ensure that you are full for longer.

It is normal for you to feel tired, grumpy, and shaky for the first few days when you start following the Atkins diet. You can stop this by drinking plenty of water, taking multivitamins and taking vitamin B12 for more energy and against the side effects of the diet.

Always consult with your doctor before starting a new diet. Also consult your doctor if there are symptoms that do not resolve, or if you continue to feel sick or unwell.

YOU CAN FOLLOW THESE RECIPES FOR GOOD DIET!

Here's a day of normal food at some stage in two levels. Phase certainly one of Atkins, the startup length, usually lasts about two weeks. Phase 4 is the long-time period upkeep level.

STUFFED CHICKEN WITH ASPARAGUS & BACON

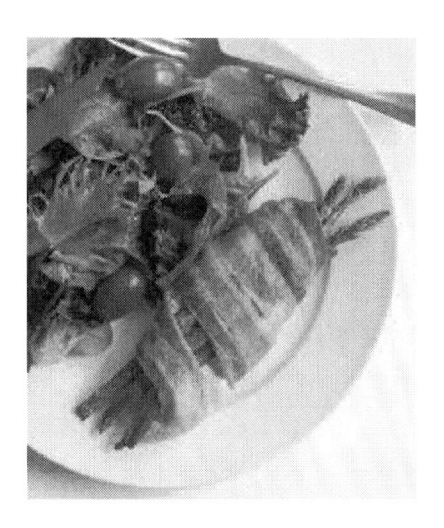

INGREDIENTS

- 8 - chicken tenders about 1 lb
- ½ - tsp salt
- ¼ - tsp pepper
- 12 - asparagus spears about .5 lb
- 8 - pieces bacon about .5 lb

INSTRUCTIONS

1. Preheat broiler to 400.

2. Lay two bits of bacon out on a heating sheet. Spot 2 fowl tenders to finish everything. Season with somewhat salt and pepper. Include 3 lances of asparagus.
3. Fold the bacon over the chicken and asparagus to safeguard every last bit of it together. Rehash.
4. Heat for 40 mins till the chicken is cooked through, the asparagus is smooth, and the bacon is fresh.

BASIL STUFFED CHICKEN BREASTS

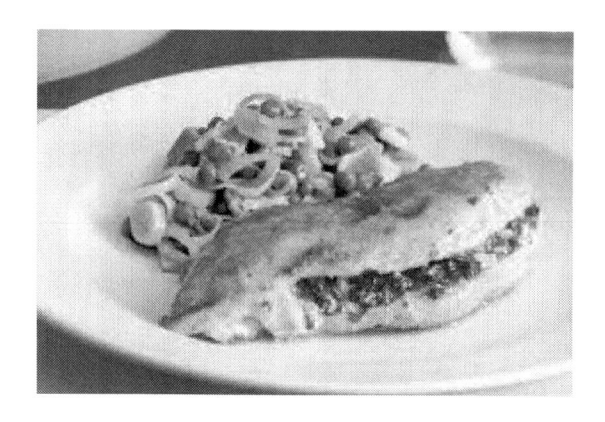

INGREDIENTS

- 2 - bone-in, skin-on chicken breasts
- 2 - tbs cream cheese
- 2 - tbs shredded cheese
- ¼ - tsp garlic paste
- 3-4 - fresh basil leaves finely chopped
- black pepper

INSTRUCTIONS

1. Preheat the broiler to 375F.
2. Make the stuffing by joining the cream cheddar, cheddar, garlic glue, basil, and dark pepper.
3. Delicately strip back the skin on one side of the chicken bosom and spot the half stuffing inside. Smooth it down and supplant the skin. Rehash for the other bit of chicken.

4. Cook on a preparing plate for 45 minutes or until the inner temperature of 165F has been come to.

5 MINUTE LOW CARB CHICKEN NUGGETS

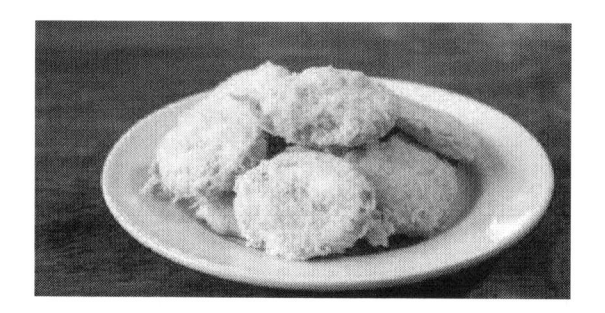

INGREDIENTS
- 2 - cups cooked chicken
- 8 - oz cream cheese
- 1 - egg
- ¼ - cup almond flour
- 1 - tsp garlic salt

INSTRUCTIONS
1. Shred chicken with an electric blender. This works high-quality with a mix of dim and chicken (or truely dull meat) that is still heat.
2. On the off danger which you are using remaining bird warm it up rather first. When the hen is destroyed encompass something is left of the fixings and mix till completely consolidated.
3. Drop scoops onto a lubed heating sheet (or use cloth paper to line it) and clean into a bit form.
4. Prepare at 350 for 12-14 min till fairly exquisite and firm.

SAUSAGE KALE SOUP WITH MUSHROOM

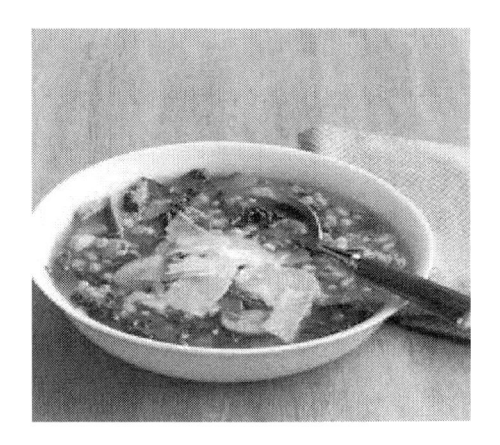

INGREDIENTS

- 29 - ounces chicken bone broth
- 6.5 - ounces fresh kale cut into bite sized pieces
- 1 - pound sausage cooked, casings removed and sliced
- 6.5 - ounces sliced mushrooms
- 2 - cloves garlic minced
- Salt & Pepper to taste

INSTRUCTIONS

1. Spot the two jars of chicken soup in expansive pot alongside two jars worth of water. Heat to the point of boiling over medium warmth.
2. Include the kale, wiener, mushrooms and garlic. Season to taste with salt and pepper.
3. Stew secured over low warmth for around 60 minutes.

BUNLESS BURGER

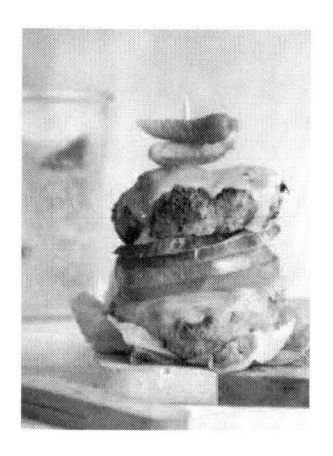

INGREDIENTS

- 1 - pound ground beef
- 1 - tablespoon Worcestershire sauce
- 1 - tablespoon Mc Cormicks Montreal Steak Seasoning
- salt & pepper

OPTIONAL

- 2 - tablespoons bacon drippings or olive oil
- 4 - ounces sliced onion

INSTRUCTIONS

1. Prep: Preheat flame broil and clean the mesh.
2. Strategy: Break up the ground hamburger and equally disseminate the Worcestershire sauce and steak flavoring and olive oil if utilizing).

3. Blend tenderly with your hands to convey the flavoring and structure into three balls. Tenderly press/pat into patties or utilize a burger press like I have imagined. On the off chance that you make a slight sorrow in the focal point of your burger, it will help keep it from puffing up in the center.
4. cook: oil the mesh. season the out of doors of the burger patties with a mild sprinkling of salt and pepper (the two aspects). flame broil for your best dimension of doneness. i really like mine really pink inside the middle. gift with your maximum cherished additional objects but do not forget to test the carbs.
5. Discretionary: For the caramelized onions… Cut the onions. Warmth 1 tablespoon of oil in a container over medium-low warmth. Whenever hot, include the onions and saute until mollified. Include 1/2 teaspoon of erythritol and cook until starting to dark colored or caramelize. This progression can take as long as 10 minutes.

WHITE LASAGNA STUFFED PEPPERS

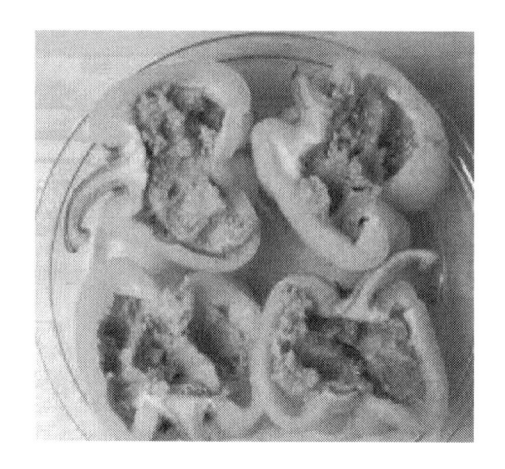

INGREDIENTS

- 2 - large sweet peppers halved and seeded
- 1 - tsp garlic salt divided
- 12 - oz ground turkey
- ¾ - cup ricotta cheese
- 1 - cup mozzarella
- 8 - cherry tomatoes

INSTRUCTIONS

1. Preheat stove to 400.
2. Put the split peppers in a preparing dish. Sprinkle with 1/4 tsp garlic salt. Partition the ground turkey between the peppers and press into the bottoms. Sprinkle with another 1/4 tsp garlic salt. Heat for 30 minutes.

3. Gap the ricotta cheddar between the peppers. Sprinkle with the rest of the 1/2 tsp garlic salt. Sprinkle the mozzarella to finish everything. Put the cherry tomatoes in the middle of the peppers, if utilizing.
4. Prepare for an extra 30 minutes until the peppers are mollified, the meat is cooked, and the cheddar is brilliant.

CREAMY BASIL BAKED SAUSAGE

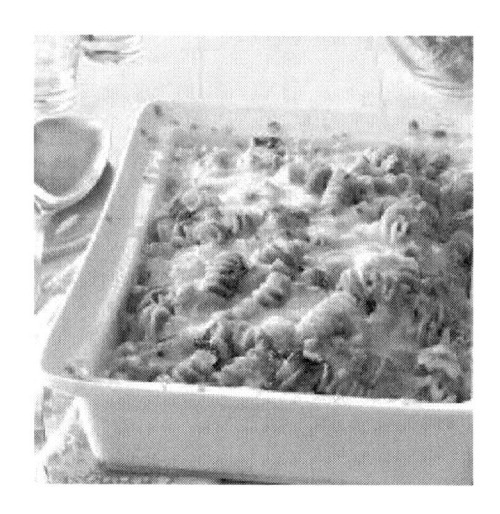

INGREDIENTS

- 3 - lb Italian sausage chicken, turkey, or pork
- 8 - oz cream cheese
- ¼ - cup basil pesto
- ¼ - cup heavy cream
- 8 - oz mozzarella

INSTRUCTIONS

1. Preheat broiler to 400. Shower a huge meal dish with the cooking splash. Put the frankfurter in the heating dish. Prepare for 30 minutes.
2. In the mean time blend together the cream cheddar, pesto, and overwhelming cream.

3. Spread the sauce over the frankfurter. Top with mozzarella. Prepare for an extra 10 minutes or until the hotdog is 160 degrees when checked with a meat thermometer.
4. Discretionary: Broil for 3 minutes to toast the cheddar to finish everything. Watch it always. It can consume effectively.

LOW CARB PORK MEDALLIONS

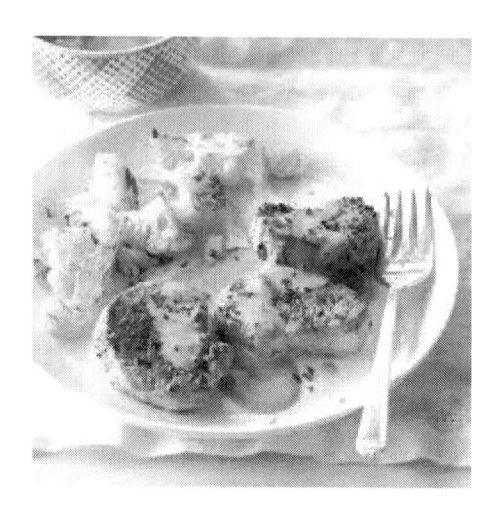

INGREDIENTS

- 1 - lb. pork tenderloin
- 3 - medium shallots (chopped nice)
- ¼ - cup oil

INSTRUCTIONS

1. Reduce the beef into half inch thick cuts.
2. hack the shallots and notice them on a plate.
3. warm the oil in a skillet
4. press every little bit of red meat into the shallots on the 2 aspects. the shallots will adhere to the pork in the event which you press solidly.
5. Spot the beef cuts with shallots into the warm oil and prepare dinner till accomplished. You will locate that a part of the

shallots will consume for the duration of cooking, but, they'll even now confer delicious taste to the beef. Panic do not as properly. Simply cook dinner the red meat until it's cooked through.

6. Present with veggies.

EASY MOZZARELLA & PESTO CHICKEN CASSEROLE

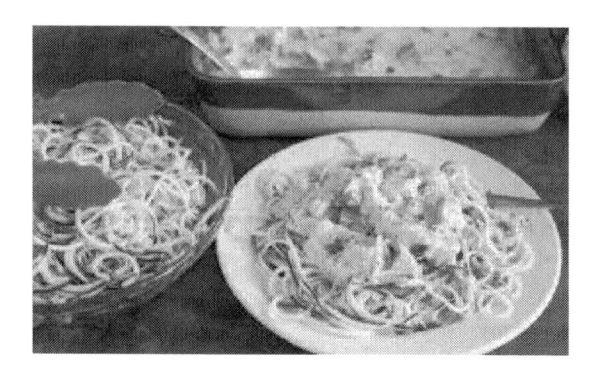

INGREDIENTS

- ¼ - cup pesto
- 8 - oz cream cheese softened
- ¼ - ½ - cup heavy cream
- 8 - oz mozzarella cubed
- 2 - lb cooked cubed chicken breasts
- 8 - oz mozzarella shredded

INSTRUCTIONS

1. Preheat stove to 400. Splash a vast meal dish with cooking shower.
2. Consolidate the initial three fixings and blend until smooth in an extensive bowl. Include the chicken and cubed mozzarella. Exchange to the goulash dish. Sprinkle the destroyed mozzarella to finish everything.

3. Prepare for 25-30 minutes. Present with zoodles, spinach, or squashed cauliflower.

EASY TACO CASSEROLE RECIPE

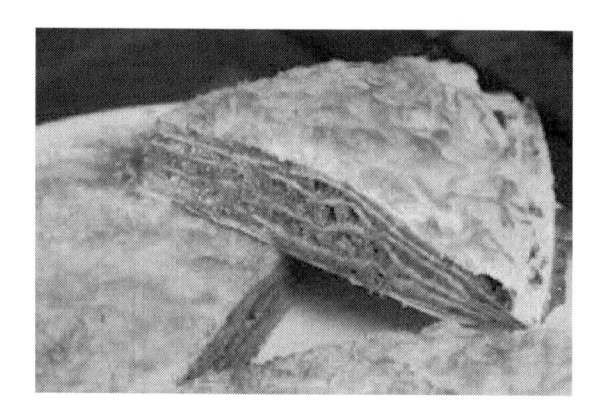

INGREDIENTS

- 1.5 to 2 - lb ground turkey or beef
- 2 - tbsp taco seasoning
- 1 - cup salsa
- 16 - oz cottage cheese
- 8 - oz shredded cheddar cheese

INSTRUCTIONS

1. Preheat stove to 400.
2. Blend the ground meat and taco flavoring in a huge meal dish. Mine is 11 x 13. Prepare for 20 minutes.
3. In the interim, combine the curds, salsa, and 1 measure of the cheddar. Put aside.
4. Take off the meal dish from the stove and cautiously channel the cooling fluid from the meat. Separate the meat into little pieces. A potato masher works incredible for this. Spread the

curds and salsa blend over the meat. Sprinkle the rest of the cheddar to finish everything.

5. Return the meal to the stove and heat for an extra 15-20 minutes until the meat is cooked completely and the cheddar is hot and bubbly.

PARMESAN CHICKEN TENDERS

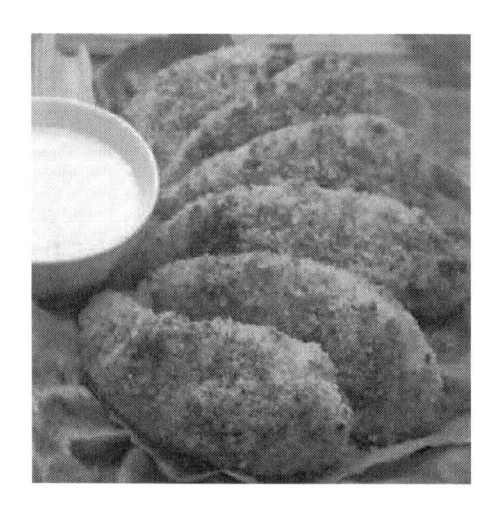

INGREDIENTS

- 1 2.5 - lb. bag chicken tenderloins
- ¾ - cup butter
- 1⅛ - cup parmesan cheese
- ¾ - tsp. garlic powder
- Salt, to taste

INSTRUCTIONS

1. Soften the margarine in a skillet and include the parmesan cheddar and garlic powder (and salt, if utilizing). Plunge the chicken in the blend and spot on a treat sheet. Prepare at 325 degrees F for 20-30 minutes (until the chicken is never again pink inside and the juices run clear). Don't overbake!
2. We have likewise utilized these for Sunday lunch. My mother set them up for chapel, at that point heated them on our stove's

"warm" setting for about 3½ hours while we were no more. Worked incredible!

BROCCOLI & CHEDDAR KETO BREAD RECIPE

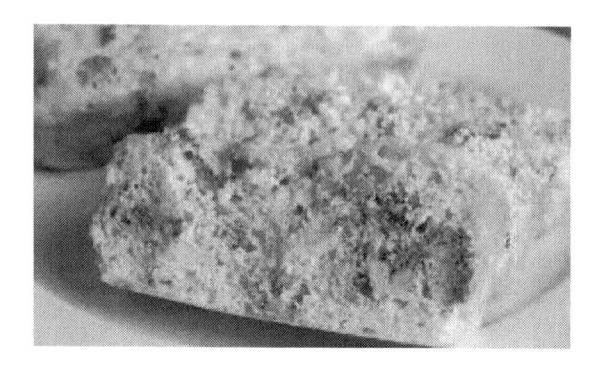

INGREDIENTS

- 5 - eggs beaten
- 1 - cup shredded cheddar cheese
- ¾ - cup fresh raw broccoli florets chopped
- 3 ½ - tbsp coconut flour
- 2 - tsp baking powder
- 1 - tsp salt

INSTRUCTIONS

1. Preheat broiler to 350. Shower a portion skillet with a cooking splash.
2. Blend every one of the fixings in a medium bowl. Fill the portion skillet.
3. Heat for 30-35 minutes or until puffed and brilliant. Cut and serve.
4. To Reheat Microwave or warmth in a lubed griddle.

BACON WRAPPED CHICKEN TENDERS WITH RANCH DIP

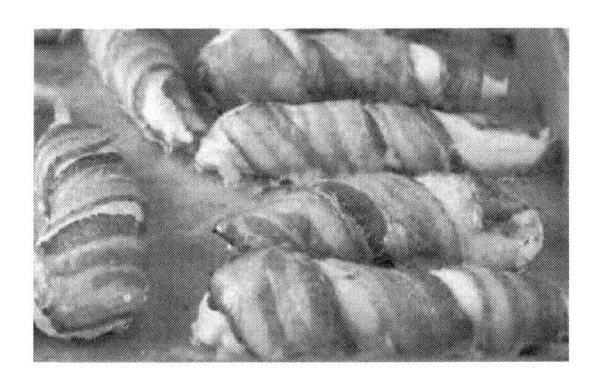

INGREDIENTS:
- 12- chicken tenderloins about 1.5 lb
- 12 - slices of bacon
- Ranch Dip Ingredients:
- 1/3 - cup sour cream
- 1/3 - cup mayo
- 1 - tsp each garlic powder onion powder, parsley, and dill
- ½ - tsp salt

INSTRUCTIONS
1. Preheat the broiler to 400.
2. Wrap every chicken delicate firmly in a bit of bacon. I extended the bacon as I folded it over the chicken.
3. Spot on a heating sheet. Prepare for 35-45 minutes until the bacon is fresh and the chicken is completely cooked.

4. In the meantime, mix together the elements for the plunge. Present with the cooked chicken.

FARMHOUSE BEANS & SAUSAGE

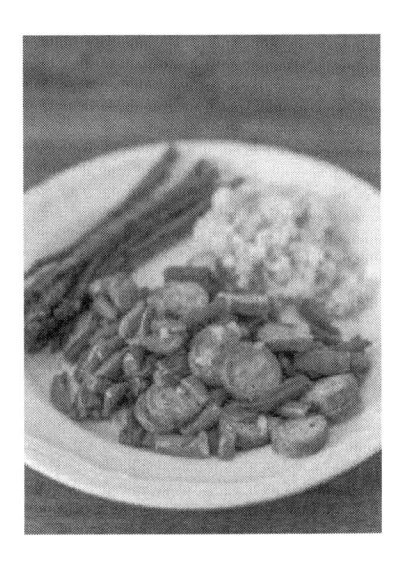

INGREDIENTS

- 2 - cups gluten-free chicken broth
- 2 16 - oz. frozen green beans
- 1 16 - oz. chicken sausage, sliced
- ½ - onion, diced
- 2 - teaspoons Herbamare
- salt & pepper to taste

INSTRUCTIONS

1. Spot all fixings in the Instant Pot. Spot top on and close ensuring the steam vent is shut.
2. Utilize manual setting and set at 6 minutes.

3. At the point when cook time is done utilize the fast discharge strategy to let off the steam.

CHICKEN AL FORNO & VODKA SAUCE WITH TWO CHEESES

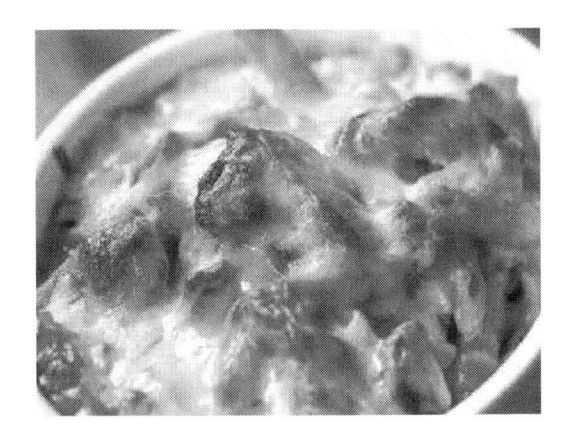

INGREDIENTS

- 2 - pounds chicken breast (cooked and cut into chunks)
- 1 ½ - cups vodka sauce jarred or homemade
- ½ - cup parmesan cheese
- 16 - oz fresh mozzarella
- fresh spinach optional

INSTRUCTIONS

1. Preheat the broiler to 400. Splash a meal dish with cooking shower. Include the cooked chicken.
2. Top with the vodka sauce, parmesan cheddar, and lumps of new mozzarella.
3. Heat until hot and bubbly. Around 25-30 minutes.
4. Discretionary: You can serve this over child spinach. The warmth from the sauce shrinks the spinach.

STUFFED PORK CHOPS – 5 INGREDIENTS

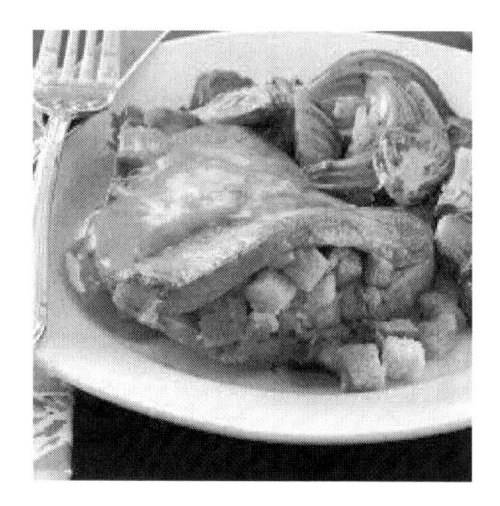

INGREDIENTS

- 12 - thin cut boneless pork chops, about 2 - 2.5 pounds
- 4 - garlic cloves
- 1 ½ - tsp salt
- 2 - cups baby spinach, about 2.5 oz
- 12 - slices provolone cheese (about 8 oz)

INSTRUCTIONS

1. Preheat the range to 350.
2. Press the garlic cloves via a garlic press into a touch bowl. add the salt and mix to consolidate. spread the garlic rub on one aspect of the beef hacks. Turn 6
3. Slashes garlic aspect down onto an expansive rimmed heating sheet. Gap the spinach between the ones 6 cleaves. Crease the

cheddar cuts down the center and placed them over the spinach. Put second pork lower over each with the garlic facet up.

4. Heat for 20 mins. Spread each pork cleave with another cut of cheddar. Back for a further 10-15 mins or till the meat is a hundred and sixty stages whilst checked with a meat thermometer.

SUPER EASY SPICY BAKED CHICKEN

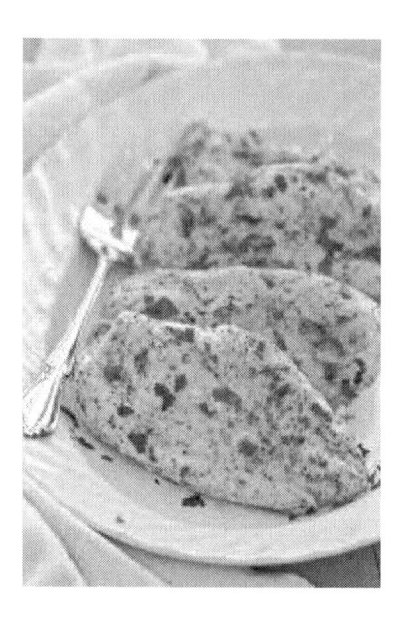

INGREDIENTS

- 4 - ounces cream cheese cut into large chunks
- ½ - cup salsa
- ½ - teaspoon sea salt
- ¼ - teaspoon black pepper freshly ground
- 1 - pound boneless, skinless chicken breasts
- 1 - teaspoon parsley finely chopped, for garnish (optional)

INSTRUCTIONS

1. Preheat stove to 350º Fahrenheit.
2. Spot cream cheddar and salsa in a little, overwhelming weight pan. Spot over low warmth and cook, blending habitually, until cream cheddar melts and joins with the salsa. Blend in ocean

salt and pepper. Expel from warmth. Mastermind chicken bosoms in a heating dish. Pour arranged cream cheddar sauce over best, covering the bosoms.

3. Prepare in the preheated stove for 40-45 minutes, or until the focus of chicken bosoms achieve 180º Fahrenheit. Take it off from a stove and sprinkle with parsley, whenever wanted, before serving.

LEMON PARMESAN BROCCOLI SOUP

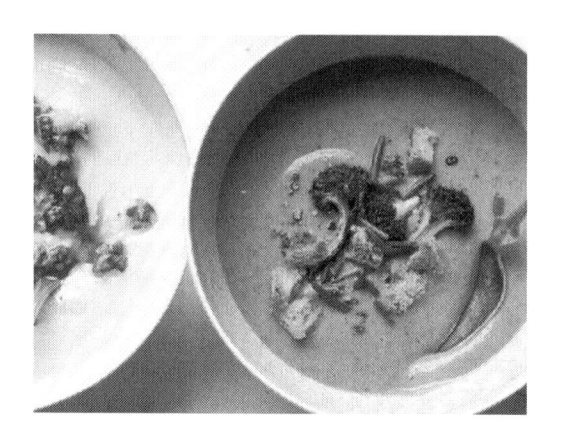

INGREDIENTS

- 2.5 to 3 - lbs of fresh broccoli florets
- 4 - cups of water
- 2 - cups unsweetened almond milk
- ¾ - cup parmesan cheese
- 2 - tbsp lemon juice

INSTRUCTIONS

1. Put the broccoli and water in a substantial pan. Spread and cook on medium high until the broccoli is delicate.
2. Save one measure of the cooling fluid and dispose of the rest.
3. Include half of the broccoli, the saved cooking fluid, and almond milk into a blender. Mix until smooth.
4. Come back to the pot with whatever is left of the broccoli. Include the parmesan and lemon squeeze and warmth until hot.

5. I didn't include salt or pepper however you might need to include a bit. Simply season to taste.

MEAT-LOVER PIZZA CUPS

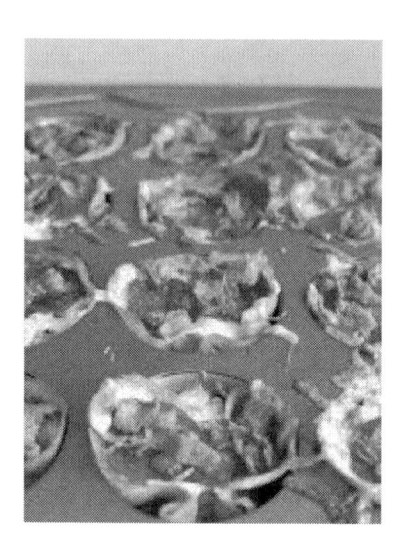

INGREDIENTS
- 12 - deli ham slices
- 1 - lb. bulk Italian sausage
- 12 - Tbsp sugar-free pizza sauce
- 3 - cups grated mozzarella cheese
- 24 - pepperoni slices
- 1 - cup cooked and crumbled bacon

INSTRUCTIONS
1. Preheat stove to 375 F. Dark colored Italian frankfurter in skillet, depleting abundance oil.
2. Line 12-container biscuit tin with ham cuts. Gap frankfurter, pizza sauce, mozzarella cheddar, pepperoni cuts, and bacon disintegrates between each container, in a specific order.

3. Prepare at 375 for 10 minutes. Cook for 1 minute until cheddar air pockets and tans and the edges of the meat garnishes look firm.
4. Take pizza containers out from biscuit tin and set on paper towel to keep the bottoms from getting wet. Appreciate promptly or refrigerate and re-heat in toaster broiler or microwave.

FRESH TOMATO BASIL SOUP

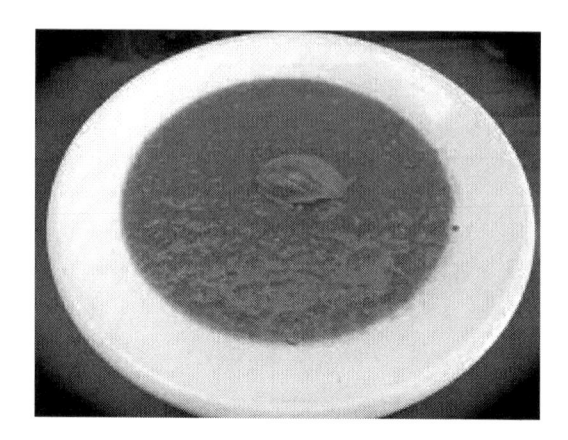

INGREDIENTS
- 5 - cups of fresh tomato puree
- 1 - stick of salted butter
- 8 - oz cream cheese
- a - handful of fresh basil leaves
- 1 - tbsp Trim Healthy Mama Gentle Sweet
- salt and pepper to taste

INSTRUCTIONS
1. Puree enough new tomatoes in a blender to measure up to five measures of puree. This was around 4 extensive tomatoes and perhaps a half quart of cherry tomatoes.
2. Turn the puree into a substantial pan and include the spread and creamy cheddar. Warmth to a stew and cook until the margarine and cream cheddar liquefy. Cautiously empty the

soup once more into the blender and include the basil (use alert mixing hot fluids - dependably vent the top) or utilize a drenching blender to puree until smooth.

RANCH YOGURT MARINADE FOR GRILLED CHICKEN

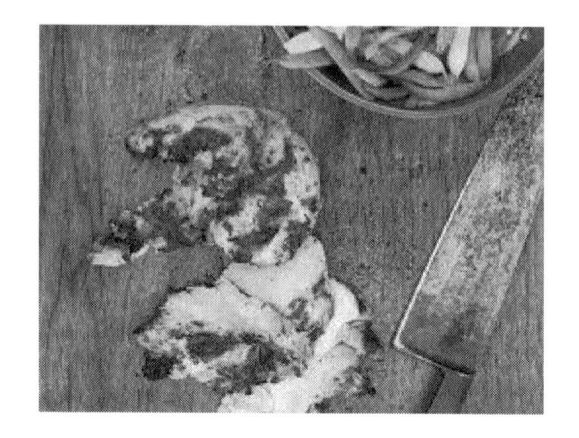

INGREDIENTS

- 1/3 - cup plain yogurt
- 1 - tbsp dill
- 1 - tbsp parsley
- 1 - tbsp onion powder
- 1 - tbsp garlic powder
- 1 - tsp salt

INSTRUCTIONS

1. Mix all ingredients in a single bowl. Add 2.5 lbs of the chicken tenders. Marinade in the fridge for at least 4 hours.

5 MINUTE 5 INGREDIENT CHEESY BACON CHICKEN

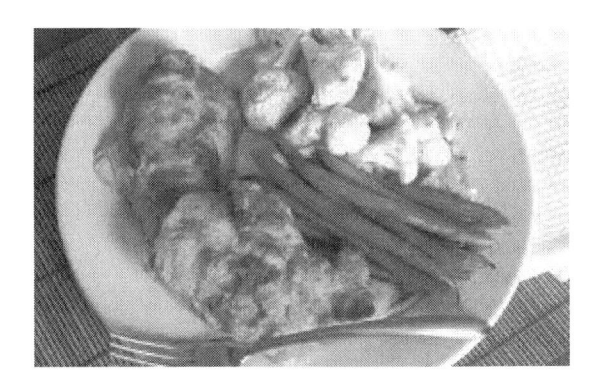

INGREDIENTS

- 5 to 6 - chicken breasts , cut in half width wise
- 2 - tbsp seasoning rub
- ½ - pound bacon , cut strips in half
- 4 - oz shredded cheddar
- sugar free barbecue sauce , optional, to serve

INSTRUCTIONS

1. Preheat stove to 400. Splash a huge rimmed preparing sheet with cooking shower.
2. Rub the two sides of chicken bosoms with flavoring rub. Top each with a bit of bacon. Prepare for 30 min on the best rack until the chicken is 160 degrees and the bacon looks firm.
3. Take plate out from the broiler and sprinkle the cheddar over the bacon. Set back in the broiler for around 10 min until the cheddar is bubbly and brilliant. Present with grill sauce.

BAKED PESTO CHICKEN

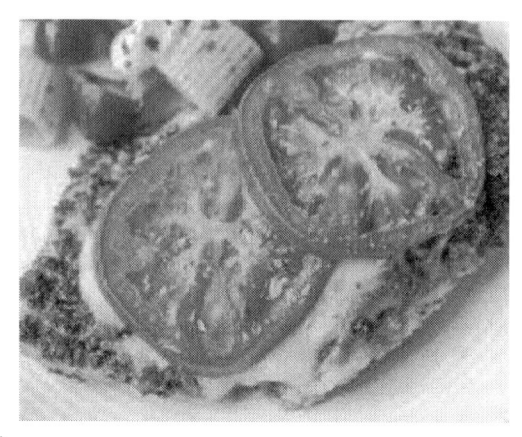

INGREDIENTS

- 4 - chicken breasts about 1.5 lb, sliced in half widthwise to make 8 pieces
- 3 - tbsp basil pesto
- 8 - oz mozzarella thinly sliced or shredded
- ½ - tsp salt
- ¼ - tsp black pepper

INSTRUCTIONS

1. Preheat stove to 350.
2. Splash making a ready dish with cooking shower. Spot chicken inside the base in a solitary layer and sprinkle with the salt and pepper. Spread the pesto on the bird. Put the mozzarella to finish everything.
3. Prepare for 35-forty five minutes till the chook is a hundred and sixty stages and the cheddar is excellent and bubbly. You can

sear it for a few minutes toward the conclusion to darker the cheddar inside the event that you want.

PIZZA CHICKEN CASSEROLE

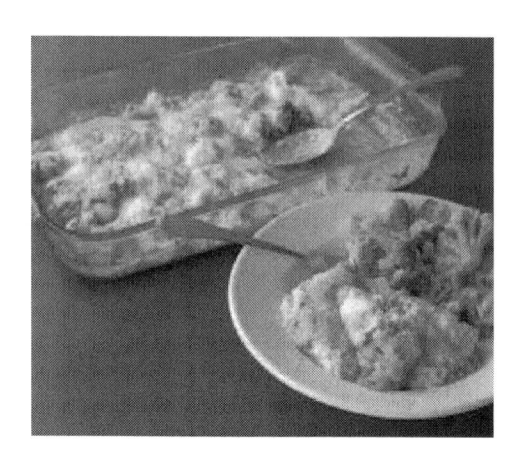

INGREDIENTS

- 1.5 to 2 - lb cooked chicken breast sliced or cubed
- 8 - oz cream cheese
- 1 - tsp dried minced garlic
- 1 - cup marinara sauce no sugar added
- 8 - oz shredded mozzarella

INSTRUCTIONS

1. Preheat oven to 350.
2. Put chicken in the backside of a 9x13 baking dish.
3. Combine cream cheese and garlic. Drop small spoonfuls onto the bird. Pour the sauce on pinnacle. Sprinkle with the shredded mozzarella.
4. Bake for 30 min or till the cheese is melted and bubbly.

KETO CAULIFLOWER AU GRATIN

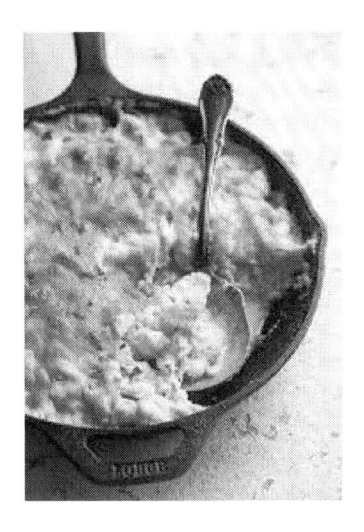

INGREDIENTS

- 1 - large head of cauliflower, trimmed and cut into florets
- 2 - small red onions, thinly sliced
- 2 - tablespoons olive oil
- 2 - tablespoons balsamic vinegar
- 1 - tablespoon granular erythritol
- ¾ - cup heavy cream
- ½ - cup finely grated parmesan
- ½ - teaspoon sea salt, more to taste
- ¼ - teaspoon black pepper, more to taste
- 1 - cup shredded gruyere or gouda cheese

INSTRUCTIONS

1. Preheat the broiler to 350°F.

2. Warmth the olive oil in a significant skillet over medium warmth. When the dish is hot, upload the onions to the field and cook dinner till delicate and sensitive, round 15 mins.
3. Include the balsamic vinegar and erythritol if utilizing, to the field with the onions, and blend to consolidate. Cook for a further 5 minutes.
4. upload cauliflower florets to the pan and blend it with the onions.
5. in a touch bowl, be part of the large cream, parmesan cheddar, salt, and pepper. pour the aggregate over great of the cauliflower.
6. sprinkle the gruyere over high-quality and prepare for 40 minutes or until the cauliflower is touchy and the splendid is first-rate dark colored and bubbly.

BOOSTED KETO COFFEE

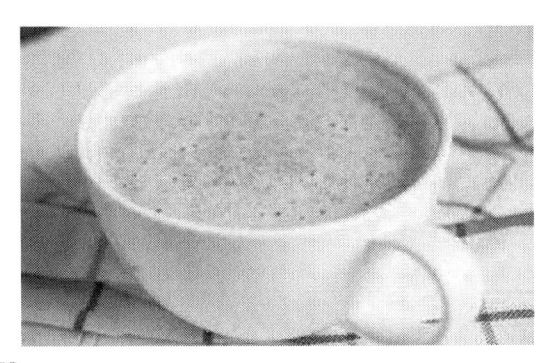

INGREDIENTS

- 8 - ounces dark roast coffee
- 1 - tablespoons butter flavored coconut oil
- 1 - scoop Keto Zone French Vanilla
- 1 - scoop Collagen Peptides
- 2 - teaspoons monk fruit sweetened caramel syrup
- Splash coconut milk

INSTRUCTIONS

1. Pour all the ingredients into a blender or milk frother and Blend till smooth and creamy. ENJOY!!

SUGAR FREE LOW CARB DRIED CRANBERRIES

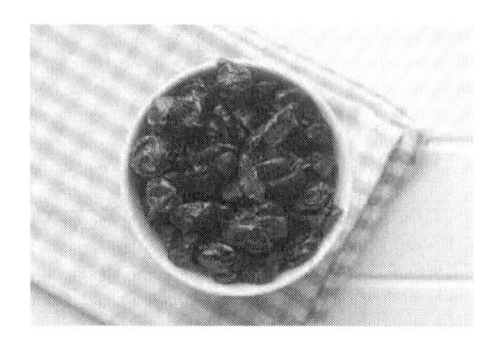

INGREDIENTS
- 2 to 12 - ounce bags fresh cranberries
- 1 - cup granular erythritol
- 3 - tablespoons avocado oil
- ½ - teaspoon pure orange extract

INSTRUCTIONS
1. Preheat the stove to 200°F. Line two rimmed preparing sheets with material paper.
2. Wash and dry the cranberries and expel any sautéed or delicate berries. Cut the cranberries into equal parts and add them to a blending bowl.
3. Include the sugar, avocado oil, and orange concentrate, if utilizing. Hurl to equitably coat the majority of the berries.
4. Line the berries in single layers over the heating sheets.
5. Heat for 3 to 4 hours, turning the racks part of the way through.

KETO HOLLANDAISE

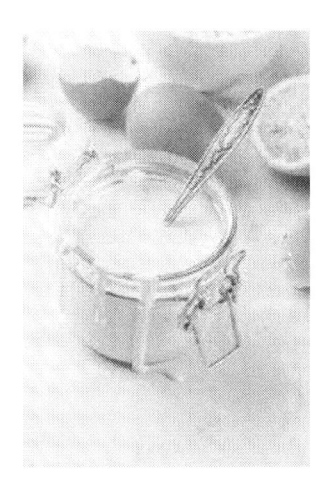

INGREDIENTS

- 4 - egg yolks
- 2 - tablespoons fresh lemon juice
- ½ - cup butter (1 stick), melted
- dash hot sauce
- pinch of cayenne pepper
- pinch of sea salt

INSTRUCTIONS

1. In a hardened metallic blending bowl, whisk the egg yolks and lemon squeeze collectively. The mixture need to get thicker and increment in quantity.
2. Warmth a pan with 1 to two crawls of water in it over medium warmth until the water is stewing. Lower the warm temperature to medium-low. Spot the bowl over quality of the

pan, ensuring that the water is not contacting the bottom of the bowl in any other case the eggs will begin to scramble. Keep whisking fast.

3. Gradually, speed within the liquefied spread until the sauce has thickened and is light and cushioned.
4. Take it out from the warm temperature and tenderly velocity within the warm sauce, cayenne pepper and ocean salt.

KETO SAUSAGE BALLS

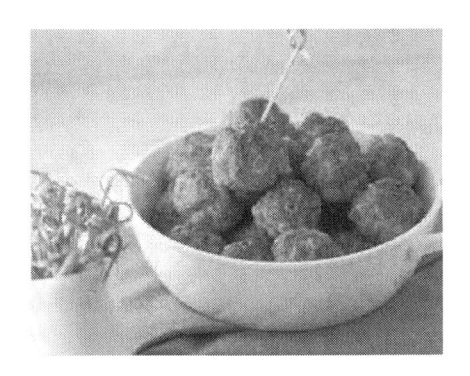

INGREDIENTS

- 1 - pound bulk Italian sausage
- 1 - cup blanched almond flour
- 1 - cup shredded sharp cheddar cheese
- ¼ - cup grated Parmesan cheese
- 1 - large egg
- 1 - tablespoon dried minced onions
- 2 - teaspoons baking powder

INSTRUCTIONS

1. Preheat the broiler to 350°F. Line a rimmed heating sheet with a wire cooling rack.
2. Join the majority of the fixings in a vast blending bowl and, utilizing your hands, blend until very much fused.
3. Structure the meat blend into 1/2 – to 2-inch meatballs, making an aggregate of 24
4. Spot the meatballs on the wire rack. Heat for 20 minutes, or until brilliant dark colored.

PORK BELLY WEDGE SALAD

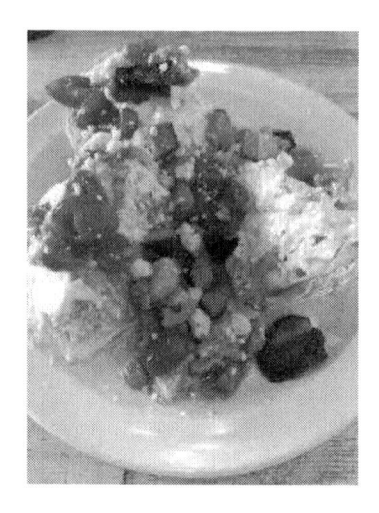

INGREDIENTS

- 1 - large head iceberg lettuce, quartered
- 1 - cup Creamy Chive Blue Cheese Dressing.
- 12 - ounces pork belly, cooked crisp and chopped
- 12 - grape tomatoes, halved
- 2 - tablespoons chopped red onion
- ¼ - cup blue cheese crumbles
- A -few sprigs fresh dill weed
- 2 - tablespoons Everything Bagel Seasoning

INSTRUCTIONS

Set each iceberg wedge on a salad plate, pinnacle with blue cheese dressing, or desired dressing of choice, after which divide the relaxation of the toppings similarly among all 4 wedges.

PICKLED RED ONIONS

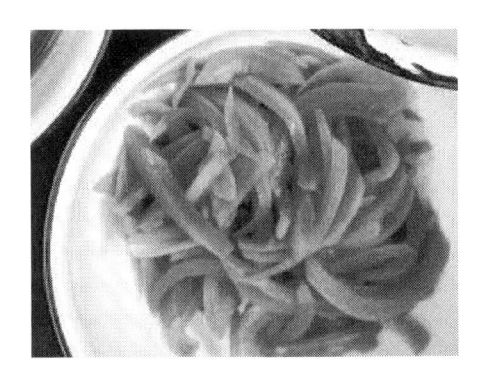

INGREDIENTS
- 1 - cup red wine vinegar
- 1 - cup apple cider vinegar
- 2 - tablespoons granular erythritol, more to taste
- 1 - teaspoons sea salt
- 2 - medium red onions, thinly sliced
- 6 - cloves garlic, peeled and halved
- 1 - teaspoon dried oregano leaves
- Pinch of red pepper flakes

INSTRUCTIONS
1. In a pan over medium warm temperature, be a part of the red wine vinegar, apple juice vinegar, erythritol, and salt. Convey to a mild bubble, blending until the erythritol and salt are damaged down.
2. Put the onions, garlic, oregano, and purple pepper portions into a 32-ounce bricklayer field.

3. Pour the fluid over satisfactory, submerging the onions and mixing inside the oregano and red pepper chips.
4. Give the box a danger to sit on the counter for 60 minutes, pinnacle and afterward refrigerate
5. save inside the fridge for as long as 2 months. you could devour them following 2 hours, however they absolutely show signs and symptoms of development and higher the more they may be within the cooler.

DAIRY FREE KETO RANCH DRESSING

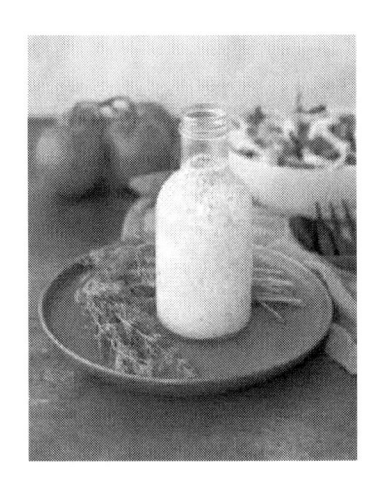

INGREDIENTS
- 1 - cup mayonnaise
- ¼ - cup water
- 2 - teaspoons chopped fresh chives
- 1 ½ - teaspoons fresh lemon juice
- 1 - teaspoon Dijon mustard
- 1 - teaspoon chopped fresh dill weed
- 1 - teaspoon chopped fresh flat-leaf parsley
- 1 - teaspoon garlic powder
- ½ - teaspoon onion powder
- ½ - teaspoon sea salt
- ½ - teaspoon black pepper

INSTRUCTIONS

1. Combine all elements together in a mason jar, cap, and shake to mix. Alternately, you may integrate all of the ingredients together in a mixing bowl, and whisk until well integrated.
2. Store within the fridge for up to 2 weeks. (If it lasts that long)

CREAMY CHIVE BLUE CHEESE DRESSING

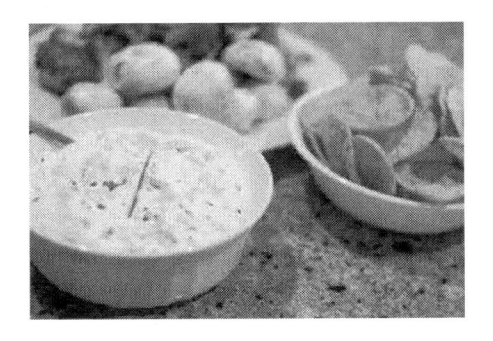

INGREDIENTS

- 1 - cup mayonnaise
- ½ - cup sour cream
- 1 - tablespoon fresh lemon juice
- 1 - teaspoon Worcestershire sauce
- 1 - teaspoon garlic powder
- ½ - teaspoon sea salt
- ½ - teaspoon black pepper
- ¾ - cup crumbled blue cheese
- ¼ - cup chopped fresh chives

INSTRUCTIONS

1. Pour all ingredients to a medium bowl or container, and mix until well combined.

BLACK BEAUTY – LOW CARB VODKA DRINK

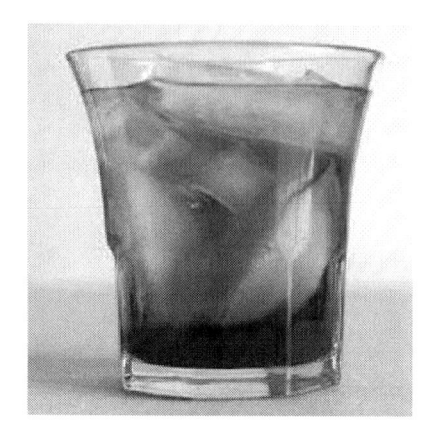

INGREDIENTS

- 2 - ounces vodka
- 5 - fresh blackberries
- ¾ - ounce fresh lemon juice (1 ½ tablespoons)
- 2 - teaspoons powdered erythritol
- ¼ - teaspoon ground black pepper
- 5 - fresh mint leaves
- Soda water

INSTRUCTIONS

1. Fill a big rocks glass with ice.
2. Consolidate the vodka, blackberries, lemon juice, erythritol, dark pepper, and mint leaves in a mixed drink shaker. Tangle until the foods grown from the ground are pounded and have discharged their juices.

3. Strain the substance of the mixed drink shaker over best of the ice.
4. Top with soft drink water and trimming with blackberries and a new mint leaf.

LOW CARB TORTILLA PORK RIND WRAPS

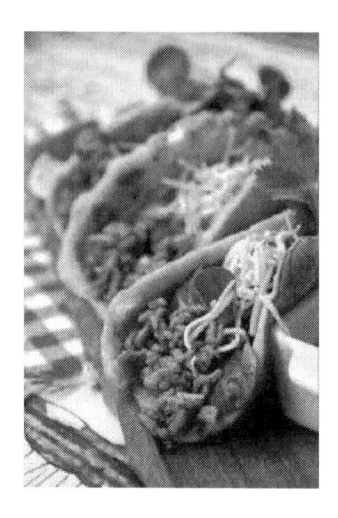

INGREDIENTS

- 4 - large eggs
- 3 - ounces pork rinds, crushed
- ½ - teaspoon garlic powder
- ¼ - teaspoon ground cumin
- ¼ - ½ - cup water
- Avocado oil or coconut oil, for the pan

INSTRUCTIONS

1. In a powerful blender or nourishment processor, consolidate the eggs, red meat skins, garlic powder, and cumin. Mix until easy and all round consolidated. Include 1/a few the water and mix over again. On the off hazard that the blend is extremely thick, preserve on along with water until it's miles the consistency of hotcake hitter.

2. Warmth an inadequate half teaspoon of oil in an 8-inch nonstick skillet over medium-low warm temperature. Twirl to coat the skillet. Include round 3 tablespoons of the participant and utilize an elastic spatula to spread it meagerly over the base of the skillet, almost to the edges.
3. Cook for approximately a second, till the bottom is beginning to darker. Release the edges and carefully flip. Cook the second facet for one greater moment or somewhere within the location.
4. Rehash with the rest of the hitter, adding oil to the skillet just as fundamental (the player spreads and chefs higher with less oil in the dish).
5. Add more water to the player as required; it'll thicken as it sits.

KETO HONEY MUSTARD CHICKEN

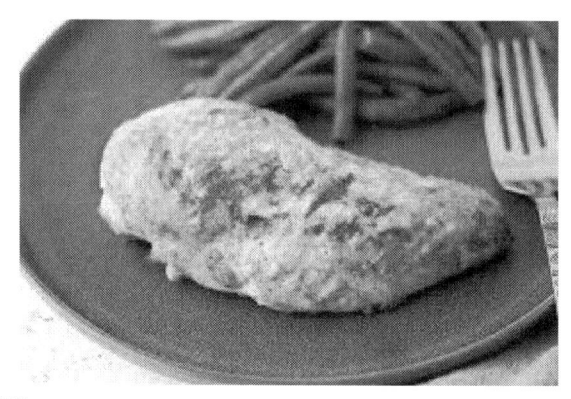

INGREDIENTS

- 4 - boneless skinless chicken breasts
- 1 - cup Keto Honey Mustard Dressing, divided
- 2 - tablespoons olive oil

INSTRUCTIONS

1. Join the chook and 1/2 degree of the nectar mustard dressing in a bowl and hurl the chicken, covering it within the dressing. Let marinate within the fridge for 60 mins, or so long as 24 hours.
2. Preheat the stove to 350°F.
3. Warmth the olive oil in a big stove-proof skillet over medium-high warm temperature. When the skillet is hot, include the chook, and dish singe, sautéing on the two sides. Around 3 to 4 minutes on each facet.

4. Pour the staying nectar mustard dressing over the bird. Move the skillet to the broiler and heat for 20 mins or until the fowl is cooked properly.

EVERYTHING BUT THE BAGEL SEASONING

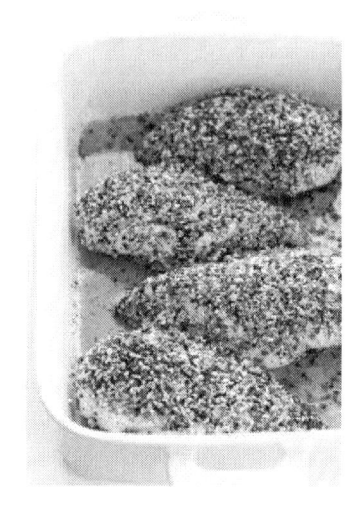

INGREDIENTS

- ¼ - cup toasted sesame seeds
- 3 - tablespoons, plus
- 1 - teaspoon poppy seeds
- 3 - tablespoons, plus
- 1 - teaspoon dried minced onions
- 3 - tablespoons, plus
- 1 - teaspoon dried garlic flakes
- 2 - tablespoons coarse sea salt

INSTRUCTIONS

1. Add all the ingredients together for mixing and store in an airtight container. Shake before using.

KETO DAIRY FREE SHAMROCK SHAKE

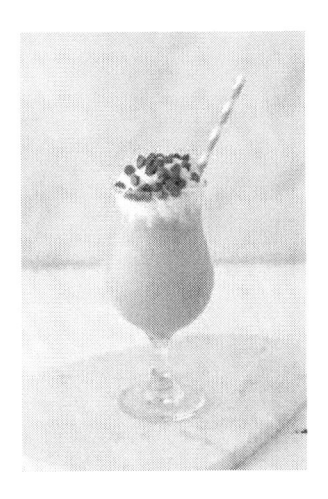

INGREDIENTS

- ½ - medium avocado
- 1 - scoop dairy free vanilla protein powder (about 30g)
- ½ - cup Silk Almond Coconut Milk
- 8 - ice cubes
- 1/8 - teaspoon peppermint extract
- 5 - drops natural green food coloring
- 2 - tablespoon coconut milk whipped cream
- 1 - tablespoon sugar-free dark chocolate chips

INSTRUCTIONS

1. Join the avocado, protein powder, almond coconut milk, ice, peppermint concentrate and sustenance shading in a blender and heartbeat until mixed and rich.
2. Top with sans dairy whipped cream and without sugar chocolate chips, if utilizing.

KETO HONEY MUSTARD DRESSING

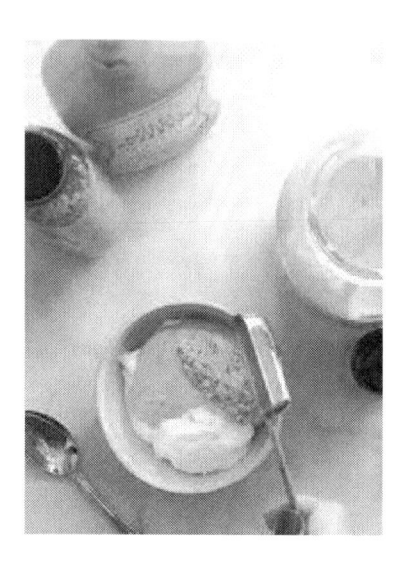

INGREDIENTS

- ½ - cup full fat sour cream
- ¼ - cup water
- ¼ - cup Dijon mustard
- 1 - tablespoon apple cider vinegar
- 1 - tablespoon granular erythritol

INSTRUCTIONS

1. Add all the ingredients in a mixing bowl or container, and mix to form. Keep in the refrigerator up to 2 weeks.

CRISPY BAKED GARLIC PARMESAN WINGS

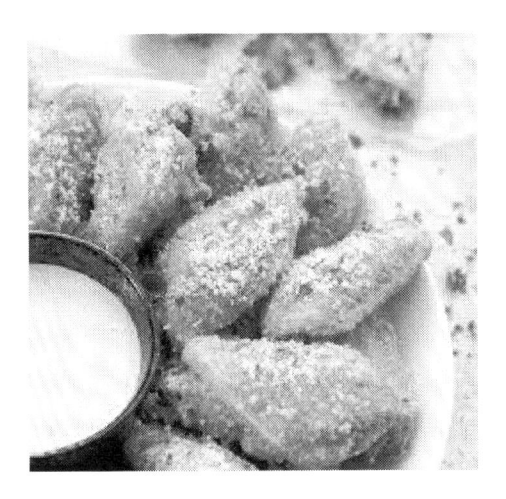

INGREDIENTS

- 2 - pounds pork baby back ribs
- 2 - tablespoons olive oil
- 1 - batch Barbecue Dry Rub

INSTRUCTIONS

1. Preheat the oven to 300°f. line a rimmed baking sheet with aluminum foil.
2. Cast off the skinny membrane from the back, or concave aspect, of the ribs. begin through reducing into the membrane with a pointy knife, then pull the skin away from the ribs. Set the ribs at the coated baking sheet.
3. Brush the olive oil lightly over the ribs. pour the dry rub over the ribs and paintings it lightly onto both sides.

4. Bake until the ribs are soft and juicy at the internal and fine and crispy at the out of doors, about 2 half of hours. Shop leftovers within the refrigerator for up to 1 week.

LOW CARB STRAWBERRY MARGARITA GUMMY

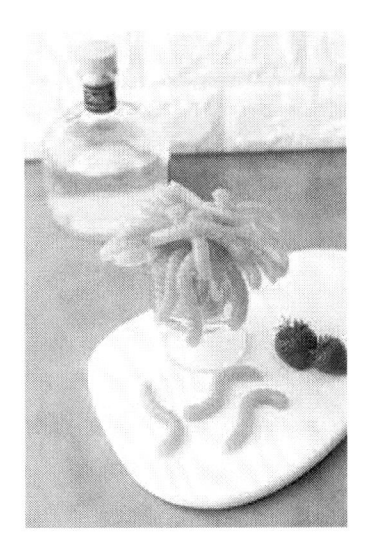

INGREDIENTS

- 10 - hulled strawberries, fresh or frozen
- 2 - ounces silver tequila
- 3 - tablespoons grass-fed gelatin collagen protein
- 2 - tablespoons powdered erythritol
- 1 ½ - ounces fresh lime juice

INSTRUCTIONS

1. Consolidate the strawberries and tequila in a blender and heartbeat until clean.
2. Pour the strawberry-and-tequila blend right into a medium pan and set over low warmth. Include the gelatin, erythritol, and lime squeeze and pace to interrupt up the gelatin and consolidate the fixings.

3. Keep on warming for round 10 minutes, whisking each every so often, till the blend ends up pourable. It will begin thick yet will land up greater slender and smoother as it warms.
4. Move the mixture to an estimating container or a bowl with a pour gush.
5. Rapidly empty the blend into the sticky trojan horse shape and exchange to the fridge.
6. Refrigerate for 10 to 15 mins, till set. Pop the sticky worms out of the shape and recognize! Store le overs within the cooler for so long as seven days.

HERBED CHICKEN AND MUSHROOMS

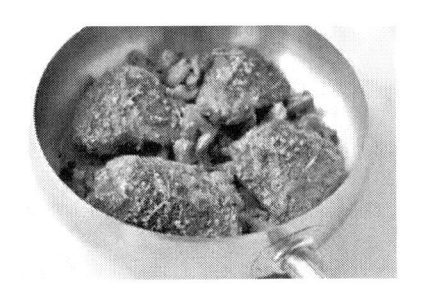

INGREDIENTS
- 8 - skin-on chicken thighs
- 2 - teaspoons sea salt
- ½ - teaspoon black pepper
- 1 - tablespoon plus 1 teaspoon dried oregano
- 1 - tablespoon plus 1 teaspoon dried thyme
- 1 - tablespoon plus 1 teaspoon dried rosemary
- 2 - tablespoons olive oil
- 8 - ounces cremini mushrooms, quartered
- 2 - cloves garlic, minced
- 1 - cup chicken stock
- 2 - tablespoons Dijon mustard
- Torn fresh parsley, optional as garnish

INSTRUCTIONS
1. Preheat the broiler to 400°F.

2. Season the chook thighs on the two facets with salt, pepper, 2 teaspoons of the oregano, 2 teaspoons of the dried thyme, and a couple of teaspoons of the dried rosemary.
3. Warmth the olive oil in an expansive cast iron skillet over medium warm temperature. Add the chook to the skillet, pores and skin aspect down. Cook for five to six minutes till the pores and skin is decent and company.
4. Flip the chicken thighs over to the alternative facet and exchange the skillet to the stove. Prepare for 15 to twenty mins, till the fowl is cooked absolutely through.
5. Move the skillet lower back to the stovetop. Expel the chook from the box, positioned apart, and spread to hold warm.
6. To a similar skillet, encompass the mushrooms and prepare dinner over medium warmth for five minutes, till they've discharged their fluid and are delicate.
7. Include the garlic, fowl inventory, Dijon mustard, and the relaxation of the seasonings and prepare dinner for an extra 3 minutes.
8. Plate the hen and pour the sauce over great. Trimming with crisp parsley, every time wanted.

PUMPKIN SPICE ROASTED PECANS

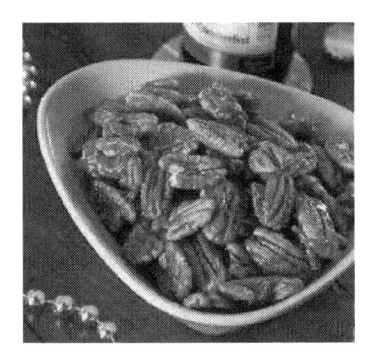

INGREDIENTS

- 2 - cups raw pecan
- 3 - tablespoons salted butter, melted
- 1 - teaspoon pure vanilla extract
- 2 - tablespoons Pumpkin Pie Spice
- 2 - tablespoons confectioners erythritol

INSTRUCTIONS

1. Preheat the broiler to 350°F. Line a rimmed preparing sheet with a silicone heating mat or material paper.
2. Include the pecans, margarine and vanilla to a blending bowl. Utilize an elastic spatula to hurl the nuts and coat them uniformly in the softened margarine.
3. Sprinkle the pumpkin pie flavor and erythritol over best. Hurl to blend in and equally coat the nuts.
4. Spread the nuts over the heating sheet in a solitary layer.
5. Heat for 12 minutes.

LOW CARB KETO BANANA NUT PROTEIN PANCAKES

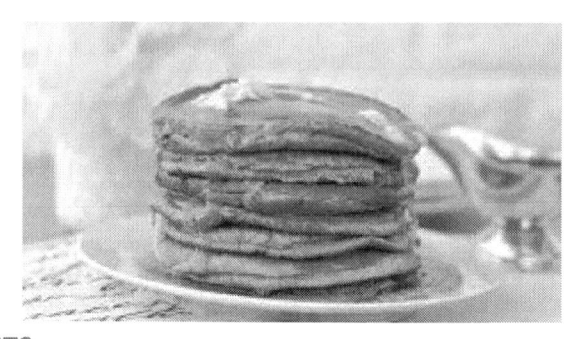

INGREDIENTS
- 2 - scoops Banana Nut Protein Powder (56 grams)
- 2 - ounces cream cheese, softened
- 4 - large pastured eggs
- 1 - teaspoon pure vanilla extract
- 2 - teaspoons baking powder
- 1 - tablespoon confectioners erythritol
- Butter for cooking

INSTRUCTIONS
1. Consolidate all fixings in a high powder blender. Heartbeat till all fixings are clean and all round joined. You may additionally want to massage the perimeters with an elastic spatula and heartbeat again to ensure the entirety is totally combined.
2. Brush a enormous non-stick skillet or frying pan field with unfold and heat over medium-low warmth. When the dish is warm, include 1/4 measure of the hitter and cook till it's far

bubbly to finish everything and fantastic darker on the base, round 3 minutes. Flip and prepare dinner the alternative aspect until it is amazing darkish colored, round 2-3 mins. Rehash this process till all the player is no more.

CHOCOLATE PEANUT BUTTER NO BAKE COOKIES

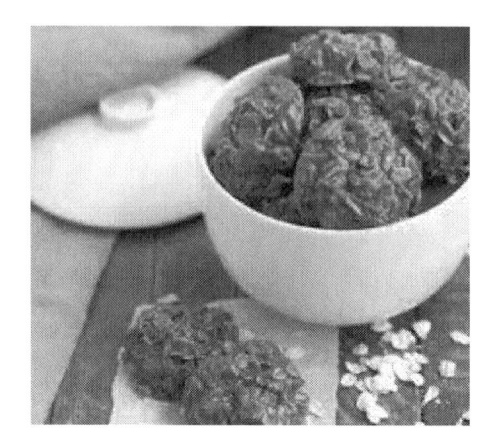

INGREDIENTS

- ¼ - cup creamy thick natural peanut butter
- ¼ - cup creamy thick natural almond butter
- 3 - tablespoons cream cheese, softened
- 2 - tablespoons salted butter, melted
- 1 - teaspoon pure vanilla extract
- 2 - tablespoons unsweetened cocoa powder
- 2 - tablespoons confectioners erythritol, more to taste
- ¾ - cup unsweetened desiccated coconut

INSTRUCTIONS

1. Set a preparing sheet with a silicone heating mat.
2. In a mixing bowl, consolidate the nutty unfold, almond margarine, and creamy cheddar. Blend till easy.
3. Include the spread, vanilla listens, cocoa powder. What's greater, erythritol. Blend until all fixings are very tons joined.

4. Utilizing an elastic spatula, overlay inside the coconut. Blend until it's far equitably disseminated during the blend.
5. Drop half to 2-inch spoonfuls (10 absolute) onto the readied heating sheet.
6. Stop for 10 mins earlier than serving.
7. Store extra items inside the cooler until prepared to eat.

LOW CARB KETO NUT FREE PIZZA CRUST

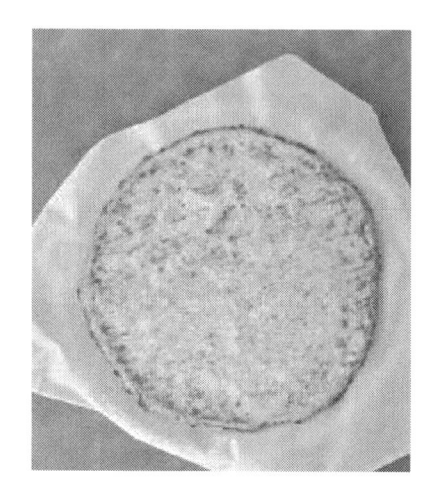

INGREDIENTS

- 4 - oz cream cheese, softened
- 2 - large eggs
- ½ - tsp garlic powder
- ½ - tsp onion powder
- ½ - tsp dried Italian seasoning
- ¼ - cup grated parmesan cheese
- 1 ¼ - cup shredded mozzarella cheese

INSTRUCTIONS

1. Preheat the broiler to 375°F Line a 12-inch pizza skillet with fabric paper. Then again you can do that on a getting ready dish, fixed with cloth paper or a silicone heating mat, or even in a lined meal dish. Work with what you've got.

2. In a blending bowl, using a hand blender, consolidate eggs, creamy cheddar, and flavoring. There will be some little clusters, but it ought to be generally clean.
3. Utilizing an elastic spatula, crease in the parmesan and mozzarella cheeses.
4. Move combo to the lined pizza box. Spread the blend out in a flimsy, even circle. For a thicker masking, make a little circle.
5. Prepare for 22 mins, flipping 12-14 minutes in. To turn it without breaking it, I like to pinnacle it with the second little bit of material paper and lift it up from the bottom, flipping it over with the brand new sheet of fabric paper under the outside, over the pizza field.

LOW CARB WHOLE30 ALMOND COCONUT MILK CREAMER

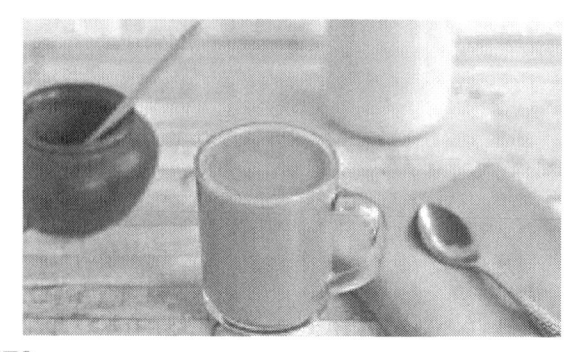

INGREDIENTS
- 2 - cups raw almonds
- 2 - cups filtered water
- 14.5 - ounce can organic coconut cream
- 2 - teaspoons pure vanilla extract

INSTRUCTIONS
1. Douse the crude almond overnight, shrouded in water. They will decrease and full. Dispose of the water.
2. Spot the almonds in an effective blender with 2 mugs crisp water, coconut cream and vanilla listen. Mix on high for 2 minutes.
3. Spot a piece strainer over a bowl or a widespread estimating container. Spot a substantial nut sack over the sifter. Empty the almond combination into the nut sack and permit it to strain through into the bowl.

4. Close the nut percent and curve across the almond mash and press. Press immovably into the strainer to separate however much milk as could moderately be predicted.
5. Keep in the refrigerator for at least seven days.

PALEO 2 MINUTE AVOCADO OIL MAYO

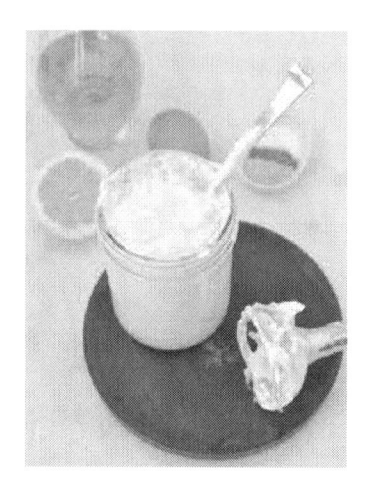

INGREDIENTS

- 2 - teaspoons lemon juice
- 1 - large egg
- ½ - teaspoon dry mustard powder
- ½ - teaspoon sea salt
- 1 - cup avocado oil

INSTRUCTIONS

1. To a tall, wide mouth artisan container include the lemon squeeze first, at that point the egg, seasonings, lastly the oil. Give the fixings a chance to rest for 20 seconds or somewhere in the vicinity.
2. Put the drenching blender the whole distance at the base of the artisan container. Turn it on fast and abandon it at the base of

the container for around 20 seconds. The mayonnaise will promptly start to set up and fill the container.

3. After the mayonnaise is practically the whole distance set, gradually pull the drenching blender towards the highest point of the container without removing the edges from the mayonnaise. At that point, gradually drive it back towards the base of the container. Rehash this stage two or multiple times until the majority of the fixings are well all around consolidated.

4. Taste and include increasingly salt, whenever wanted.

KETO SAUSAGE AND EGG BREAKFAST SANDWICH

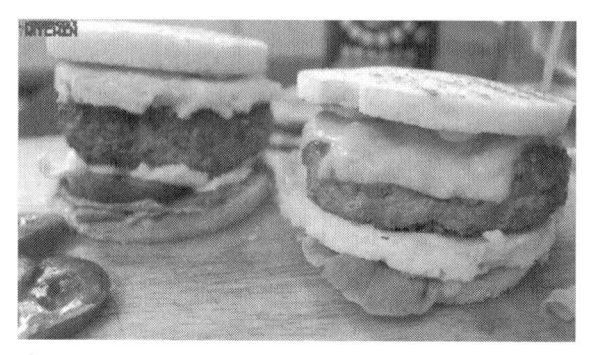

INGREDIENTS

- 1 - tbsp butter
- 2 - large eggs
- 1 - tbsp mayonnaise
- 2 - sausage patties, cooked
- 2 - slices sharp cheddar cheese
- a - few slices of avocado

INSTRUCTIONS

1. Warmth the margarine in a huge skillet over medium warmth. Spot delicately oiled artisan container rings or silicone egg molds into the dish.
2. Split the eggs into the rings and utilize a fork to break the yolks and tenderly whisk. Spread and cook for 3-4 minutes or until eggs are cooked through. Take off the eggs from the rings.
3. Spot one of the eggs on a plate and best it with half of the mayonnaise. Top the egg with one of the wiener patties.

HOT CRAB AND ARTICHOKE DIP

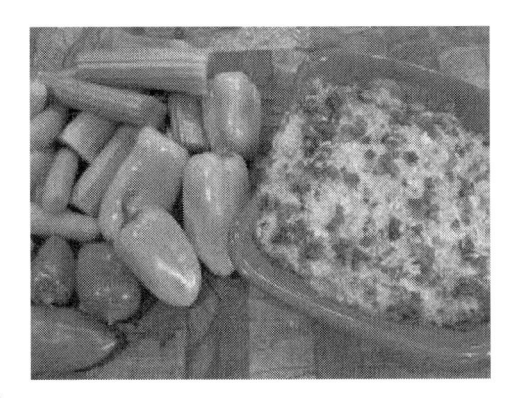

INGREDIENTS

- 8 - oz lump crab meat
- 14 - oz can artichoke hearts, drained and chopped
- 1 - cup sharp cheddar cheese, shredded
- ¾ - cup Parmesan cheese, shredded, divided
- ¾ - cup sour cream
- ½ - cup mayonnaise
- 3 - green onions, chopped
- 3 - large cloves garlic, minced
- 1 - tsp garlic powder
- 1 - tsp onion powder

INSTRUCTIONS

1. Preheat stove to 350°
2. In an extensive blending bowl, join crab meat, artichoke hearts, cheddar, ½ container Parmesan cheddar, acrid cream,

mayonnaise, green onion, garlic, garlic powder, and onion powder. Blend until all fixings are all around fused.

3. Move crab blend into a shallow preparing dish.
4. Prepare for 30 minutes on top rack.
5. Sprinkle remaining ¼ container Parmesan cheddar over the best and sear on high 3-5 minutes.

ROASTED RED PEPPER GARLIC AIOLI

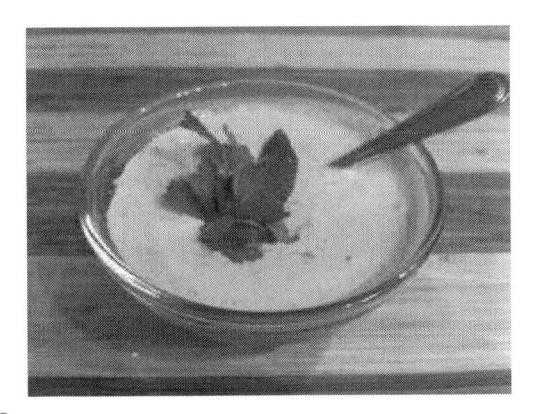

INGREDIENTS

- ¾ - cup mayo
- 6 - cloves garlic, minced
- 2 - tablespoons fresh lemon juice
- ½ - cup chopped roasted red peppers
- a - few sprigs fresh flat-leaf parsley
- ¼ - teaspoon sea salt, more to taste
- pinch of black pepper, more to taste

INSTRUCTIONS

1. Place all substances in a food processor or excessive-powered blender and pulse till well blended and smooth.
2. Refrigerate for as a minimum 30 minutes before serving.

LOW CARB TURKEY CLUB PINWHEELS

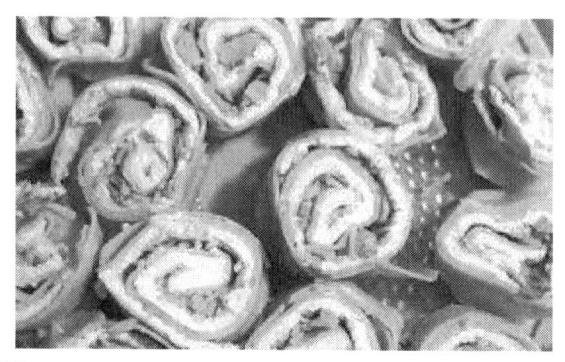

INGREDIENTS

- 2 - Large Low Carb Tortillas
- 12 - Slices Deli Turkey
- 6 - Strips Thick Cut Bacon – Cooked Crisp
- 4 - oz. Roasted Red Peppers
- 2 - oz. Cream Cheese – Softened
- 2 - Tbs. Ranch Dressing
- 1 - Medium Avocado – Peeled, Pitted and Sliced

INSTRUCTIONS

1. Join cream cheddar and farm dressing and separation similarly between the two tortillas. Spread equitably, covering one entire side of every tortilla.
2. Top every tortilla with half of the turkey, bacon, broiled red peppers, and avocado cuts.
3. Move up firmly, being mindful so as not to press the fixings out of the sides.

4. Wrap firmly in cling wrap and refrigerate for 30 minutes or until the wraps are firm enough to cut.

LOW CARB CAULIFLOWER RICE MUSHROOM RISOTTO

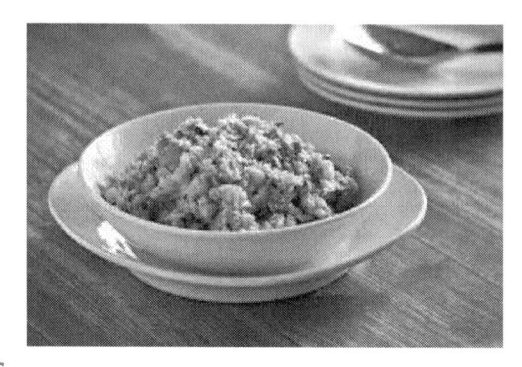

INGREDIENTS

- 2 - tablespoons butter
- 2 - tablespoons olive oil
- 6 - cloves garlic, minced
- 1 - small onion, diced
- 1 - large shallot, minced
- 8 - ounces cremini mushrooms, thinly sliced
- 2 - cup chicken stock, divided
- 4 - cups riced cauliflower
- 1 - cup heavy cream
- ½ - cup grated Parmesan cheese
- 2 - tablespoons chopped fresh flat-leaf parsley
- Sea salt and black pepper, to taste

INSTRUCTIONS

1. In a big sauté container, heat the spread and olive oil over medium warmth. To the skillet, including the garlic, onion, and

shallot. Sauté until the onions are delicate and translucent and the garlic is fragrant. Around 5 minutes.

2. To the skillet, including the mushrooms and 1 glass chicken stock. Sauté until mushrooms are delicate and have discharged their fluid. Around 5 minutes.
3. Include the cauliflower and remaining 1 measure of chicken stock and blending much of the time, sauté for 10 minutes.
4. Lessen the warmth to low, mix in the overwhelming cream, Parmesan cheddar, parsley, salt, and pepper. Let stew for 10 to 15 minutes to thicken.

KETO CHILI DOG POT PIE CASSEROLE

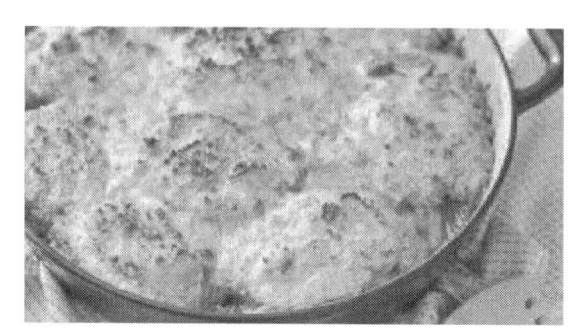

INGREDIENTS

- 1 - batch Slow Cooker Kickin' Chili
- 2 - tbsp butter
- 8 - grass-fed beef hot dogs, sliced
- 1 ½ - cups shredded sharp cheddar cheese
- 1 ½ - cups shredded mozzarella cheese
- 1 - batch Low Carb Cheddar Biscuit Dough (minus the sausage)

INSTRUCTIONS

1. Set up the stew early. You can radically decrease the cook time of this formula by changing over the bean stew to a stovetop formula.
2. Warmth the spread in a huge ovenproof skillet over medium warmth. When the spread is liquefied and the dish is hot, add the cut wieners to the container and cook until they have a decent singe on them.
3. Pour the whole clump of bean stew over the cooked wieners.

4. Blend the cheddar and mozzarella cheeses and sprinkle them over best of the bean stew.
5. Set up the scone mixture as indicated by the headings (less the hotdog)
6. Preheat broiler to 350°
7. Drop vast scoops of the bread mixture over the meal.
8. Heat for 30 minutes or until the bread topping is brilliant darker.

LOW CARB CROCK POT PIZZA CASSEROLE

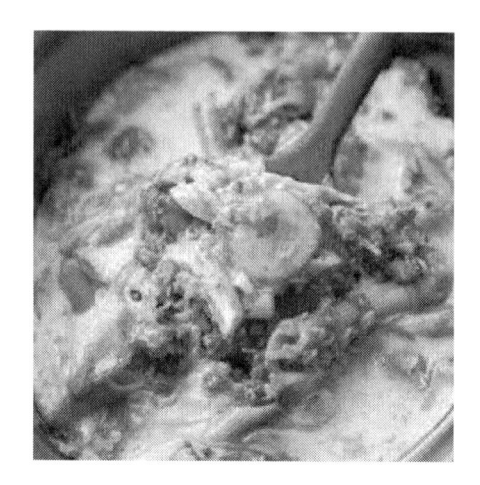

INGREDIENTS

- 1 - pound ground pork
- 1 - pound ground beef
- 2 - tablespoon pizza seasoning
- 1 - cup diced peppers onions, olives, mushrooms or other pizza toppings
- 1 - can diced tomatoes drained
- 1 - jar pizza sauce
- 2 - cups shredded mozzarella cheese
- 30 - pepperoni slices

INSTRUCTIONS

1. Dark colored ground meats with seasonings with pizza flavoring over medium warmth.

2. Include veggies or pizza garnishes other than pepperoni for 2-3 minutes till dampness is cooked out. Blend in depleted diced tomatoes.
3. Pour meat into the goulash simmering pot. Spread out over the slow cooker.
4. Pour sauce over meat and spread out equitably.
5. Sprinkle equitably with cheddar.
6. Top with pepperonis. You have two additional items - appreciate inspecting.
7. Put the top on and cook for two hours on high or 3-4 hours on low.

LOW CARB TACO CASSEROLE

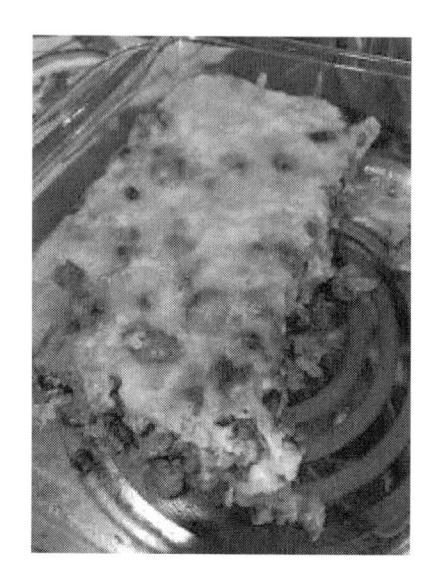

INGREDIENTS

- 1 - pound ground beef
- ¼ - cup chopped onion
- 1 - jalapeno minced
- 1 - packet taco seasoning or homemade
- ¼ - cup water
- 2 - ounces cream cheese
- ¼ - cup salsa
- 4 - eggs
- 1 - tablespoon hot sauce
- ¼ - cup heavy whipping cream
- ½ - cup grated cheddar
- ½ - cup grated pepperjack cheese

INSTRUCTIONS

1. Preheat broiler to 350 degrees. Shower an 8x8 preparing dish with the non-stick splash.
2. Dark colored the ground hamburger in a huge skillet over medium warmth.
3. Add the onions and jalapeno to the meat and cook until onion is translucent. Channel any oil.
4. Mix in the taco flavoring and water and cook for 5 minutes.
5. Include the cream cheddar and salsa and mix to join.
6. Break the eggs in a medium combining bowl and race with the hot sauce and overwhelming cream.
7. Pour the meat blend into the readied preparing dish and best with the egg blend.
8. Sprinkle with cheddar and heat for 30 minutes or until eggs are set.
9. Cool 5 minutes before cutting and serving.

EASY LOW CARB BREAKFAST CASSEROLE

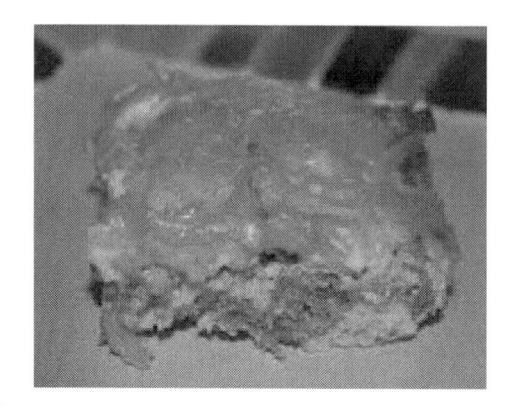

INGREDIENTS

- 1 - pound Ground breakfast sausage
- 1 - tablespoon Garlic minced
- 2 - cups Bell peppers diced
- ½ - cup Yellow onion diced
- 3 - cups Spinach chopped
- 12 - Eggs
- 1/8 - teaspoon each Salt and pepper or to taste
- ½ - cup Cheddar cheese shredded

INSTRUCTIONS

1. Preheat broiler to 350 degrees F and set up a preparing dish with non-stick cooking shower and put aside.
2. Ground and cook wiener in a skillet until completely cooked. Include garlic, peppers, and onions to the skillet and sauté with

a hotdog for 2 minutes. Spot this in your readied heating dish. Include cleaved spinach top.

3. In a different bowl whisk eggs with salt and pepper. Pour egg wash over vegetables in the heating dish and tenderly blend to ensure eggs are covering the whole dish. Top with cheddar and prepare for 45 minutes or until a fork can tell the truth and eggs are cooked entirely through.

CHEESY CHICKEN AND BROCCOLI CASSEROLE

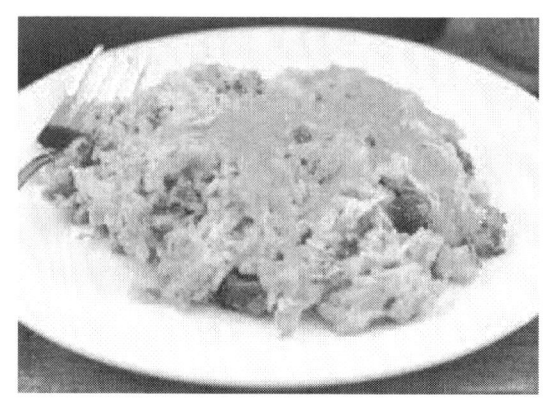

INGREDIENTS

- 3 - Cups Shredded Cooked Chicken Breast
- 5 - Cups Chopped Fresh Broccoli
- 8 - oz. Cream Cheese Softened
- 1 - Cup Sour Cream
- ½ - Cup Mayonnaise
- 1 - Teaspoon Garlic Salt
- 1 - Teaspoon Onion Powder
- ½ - Teaspoon Basil
- ¼ - Teaspoon Smoked Paprika
- ¼ - Teaspoon Rosemary
- ¼ - Teaspoon Thyme
- 1 - Cup Shredded Cheese I used Mozzarella, but you can use any kind

INSTRUCTIONS

1. Preheat broiler to 350.

2. In a vast blending bowl, consolidate all fixings aside from destroyed cheddar.
3. Pour blend into a 9x13 skillet and best with 1 container destroyed cheddar.
4. Prepare for 30-35 minutes, or until cheddar just begins to dark colored.

SPINACH AND MUSHROOM BREAKFAST CASSEROLE

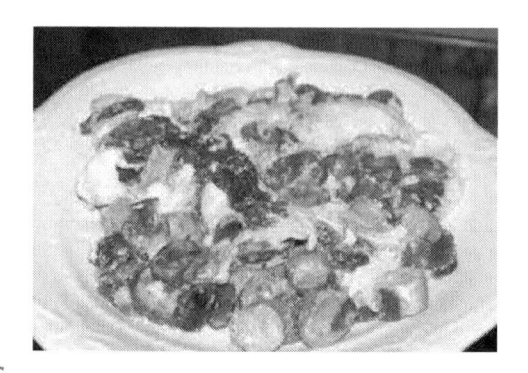

INGREDIENTS

- 12 - ounce bag fresh baby spinach
- 1/2 - lb. mushrooms sliced
- 3 - green onions sliced
- 1 - medium onion chopped
- 2 - cloves garlic minced
- 6 - eggs beaten
- 5 - Tablespoons unsalted butter divided
- 16 - oz. cottage cheese
- 12 - ounces sharp cheddar cheese grated
- 1 - teaspoon kosher salt
- ½ - teaspoon black pepper

INSTRUCTIONS

1. Pre-heat broiler to 350* F. Utilizes 1 Tablespoon spread to grease 13" X nine" heating dish.

2. Warmth 4 Tablespoons margarine in an intensive skillet or sauté container, and sauté onions, mushrooms, and garlic for 3-four of mins until onions are translucent and mushrooms are delicate.
3. Include spinach, a group at any given second, and sauté. Spread skillet and allow spinach decrease, round five mins.
4. Give cool, a risk to empty abundance fluid, and hack all the greater finely every time desired.
5. In a special bowl, whisk eggs, curds, cheddar, and salt and pepper. Include cooked spinach and mushroom combination.
6. Blend properly and fill making ready dish.
7. Heat for 45-50 mins or until fine is tremendous darkish coloured and attention is finished.

ALFREDO SAUCE RECIPE

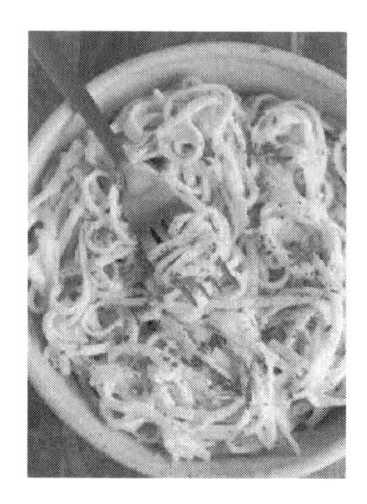

INGREDIENTS

- 2 - tablespoons Unsalted Butter Stick
- 1 ½ - cups Heavy Cream
- ½ - cup Parmesan Cheese (Grated)
- 4 - oz Romano Cheese
- 1/8 - tsp Black Pepper
- 1/8 - tsp Nutmeg (Ground)

INSTRUCTIONS

1. Liquefy margarine in a medium pot over medium warmth. Include cream and stew until diminished to 1 glass, around 10 minutes. Mesh Parmesan and Romano cheeses.
2. Pour from warmth; blend in Parmesan, Romano, pepper and nutmeg until the cheeses have softened and sauce is smooth.
3. Serve promptly.

ALMOND & COCONUT FLOUR MUFFIN IN A MUG

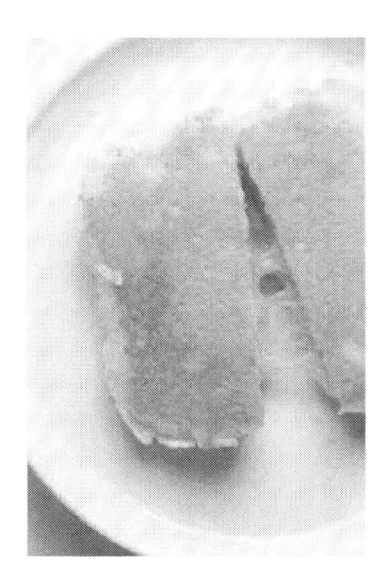

INGREDIENTS

- 2 - tbsps Almond Meal Flour
- 1/3 - tbsp Organic High Fiber Coconut Flour
- 1 - teaspoon Sucralose Based Sweetener (Sugar Substitute)
- ½ - tsp Cinnamon
- ¼ - tsp Baking Powder (Straight Phosphate, Double Acting)
- 1/8 - tsp Salt
- 1 - large Egg
- 1 - tsp Extra Virgin Olive Oil

INSTRUCTIONS

1. Spot every dry fixing in an espresso cup. Blend to consolidate.
2. Include the egg and oil. Mix until completely consolidated.

3. Microwave for 1 minute. Utilize a blade if important to help cut the biscuit off from the glass, cut, margarine, eat.

CAPRESE SNACK

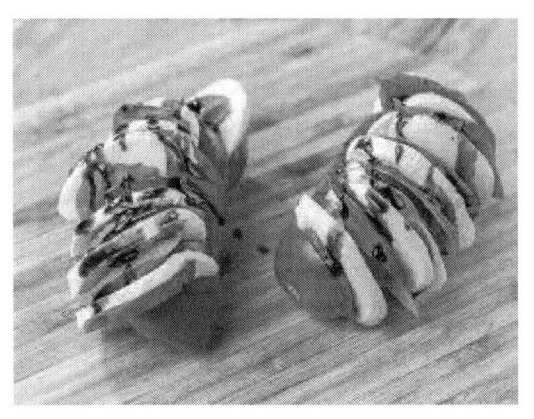

INGREDIENTS

- 8 - oz. cherry tomatoes
- 8 - oz. mozzarella, mini cheese balls
- 2 - tbsp green pesto
- salt and pepper

INSTRUCTIONS

1. Cut the tomatoes and mozzarella balls fifty-fifty. Include pesto and blend.
2. Salt and pepper to taste.

ORIENTAL RED CABBAGE SALAD

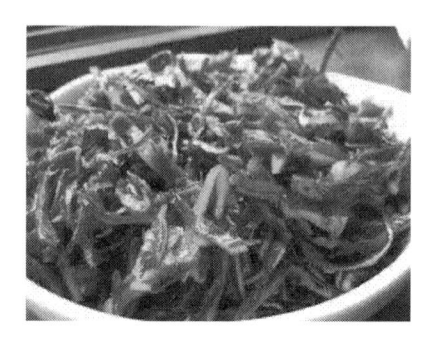

INGREDIENTS

- 30 - oz. red cabbage
- 4¼ - oz. butter
- 1 - tsp salt
- ¼ - tsp ground black pepper
- 1 - cinnamon stick
- 1 - tbsp red wine vinegar
- 1 - orange, juice and zest
- 2 - tbsp fresh dill, chopped

INSTRUCTIONS

1. Shred the cabbage finely, in a perfect world with a mandolin slicer or in a nourishment processor.
2. Broil in a spread on medium high for 10– 15 minutes. Sear the cabbage delicately until delicate and sparkly - not very dark colored.

3. Salt and pepper. Include cinnamon, vinegar and squeezed the orange. Let stew for 5-10 minutes.
4. Include pizzazz and dill towards the end or when serving.

SALAD IN A JAR

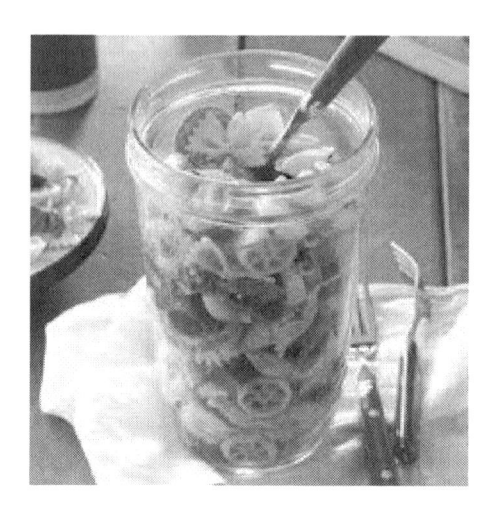

INGREDIENTS

- 4 - oz. smoked salmon or rotisserie chickens
- 1/6 - oz. leafy greens
- 1/6 - oz. cherry tomatoes
- 1/6 - oz. red bell peppers
- 1/6 - oz. cucumber
- ½ - scallion
- 4 - tbsp mayonnaise or olive oil

INSTRUCTIONS

1. Shred or hack vegetables of your decision. In the first place, put dim verdant greens, for example, spinach or arugula at the base of the container. Ice shelf lettuce or romaine works as well. Green and red cabbage give a crisp crunch. Hacked broccoli or cauliflower additionally works extraordinarily.

2. Include cut onion rings, destroyed carrot, avocado, distinctive ringer peppers and tomato in layers.
3. We have finished our serving of mixed greens with smoked salmon and barbecued chicken, yet you can obviously utilize your very own most loved protein, bubbled eggs, mackerel or canned fish or any sort of virus cuts you need. Olives, nuts, seeds, and cheddar 3D squares are extraordinary tasty increments.
4. To feel fulfilled, you might need to include a liberal measure of dressing or mayonnaise that you store in a different little container or jug and include directly before serving.

COLESLAW

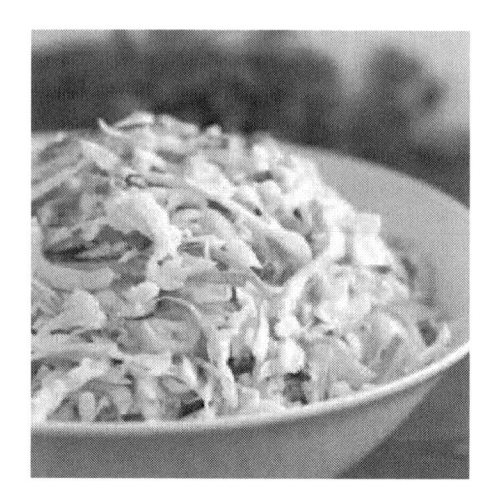

INGREDIENTS

- ½ - lb green cabbage
- ½ - lemon, the juice
- 1 - tsp salt
- ½ - cup mayonnaise
- 1 - pinch fennel seeds (optional)
- 1 - pinch pepper
- 1 - tbsp Dijon mustard

INSTRUCTIONS

1. Take off the center and shred the cabbage utilizing a nourishment processor, mandolin or sharp cheddar slicer.
2. Spot the cabbage in a medium-sized bowl.
3. Include salt and lemon juice.

4. Mix and permit take a seat for 10 mins to offer the cabbage a chance to reduce rather. Dispose of any abundance of fluid.
5. Blend cabbage, mayonnaise, and discretionary mustard.
6. Season to taste.

ASPARAGUS AND LEEK SOUP

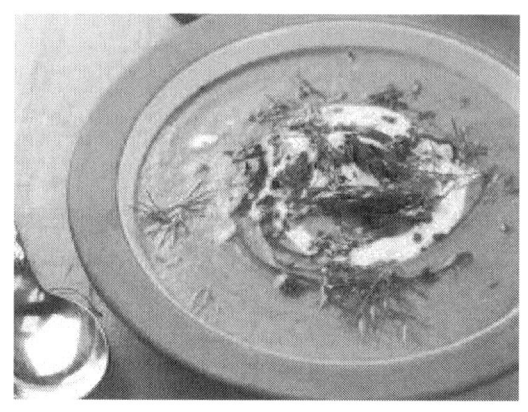

INGREDIENTS

- 2 - tablespoons Unsalted Butter Stick
- 1 - each Leeks
- ¾ - lb Asparagus
- 1 - tsp Garlic
- 1 14.5 - oz can Chicken Broth, Bouillon or Consomme
- 1/3 - cup Heavy Cream

INSTRUCTIONS

1. Liquefy margarine in an extensive pot over medium-high warmth. Clean the leeks and bones the white and a portion of the green tops. Hack asparagus into 1-2 inch pieces.
2. Add to leeks to the container and sauté for 3 minutes. Include asparagus and cook 1 minute more. Include garlic and sauté for 30 additional seconds.
3. Add stock to pot and heat to the point of boiling.

4. Lower warmth, spread and stew 8 to 10 minutes, until asparagus is delicate.
5. Blend in cream, and season with salt and naturally ground dark pepper. Mix soup in a nourishment processor or blender until smooth.
6. Come back to pot to warm through before serving (if important). Season with extra salt and newly ground dark pepper to taste.

ASIAN LOBSTER SALAD

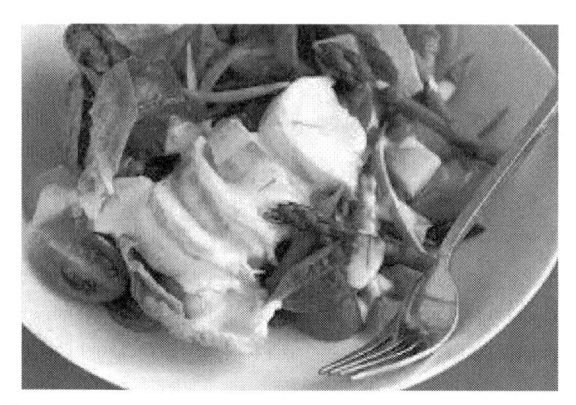

NGREDIENTS

- ¾ - lb Northern Lobster
- 2 - cup, shreddeds Chinese Cabbage (Bok-Choy, Pak-Choi)
- ½ - small Sweet Red Pepper
- 4 - medium (4-1/8" long) Scallions or Spring Onions
- 1 - tbsp Dried Whole Sesame Seeds
- 2 - tbsps Sodium and Sugar Free Rice Vinegar
- 2 - tbsps Tamari Soybean Sauce
- 1 - tsp Ginger
- 1 - tbsp Canola Vegetable Oil
- 1 - tsp Sesame Oil

INSTRUCTIONS

1. For the plate of mixed greens: In an expansive serving bowl, join lobster, cabbage, ringer pepper, scallions, and sesame seeds.

2. For the dressing: In a little bowl, whisk the rice vinegar, Tamari soy sauce, ground ginger, and the canola and sesame oils together.
3. Pour dressing over the serving of mixed greens and hurl delicately to coat. Season with crisp ground dark pepper and salt.

SIAN-STYLE COLESLAW

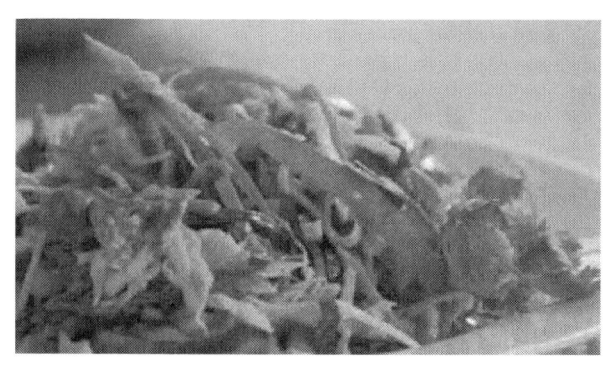

INGREDIENTS

- 1 - cup, chopped Snowpeas (Pea Pod)
- 1 - large (7-1/4" to 8-1/2" long) Carrots
- 12 - oz Chinese Cabbage (Bok-Choy, Pak-Choi)
- 2 - tablespoons Extra Virgin Olive Oil
- 1 - tbsp Toasted Sesame Oil
- 2 - tbsps Sodium and Sugar Free Rice Vinegar
- 1 - tbsp Tamari Soybean Sauce
- 2 - tsps Ginger
- 1 - tsp No Calorie Sweetener

INSTRUCTIONS

1. Shredd cabbage at that point place in a vast bowl. Mesh the carrot into a cabbage. Blend in daintily cut snow peas.
2. In a little bowl, blend oils, vinegar, tamari, ginger, and sugar substitute.

3. Pour dressing over a plate of mixed greens; hurl to coat. Season to taste with salt.

2 INGREDIENT LOW CARB CREPES

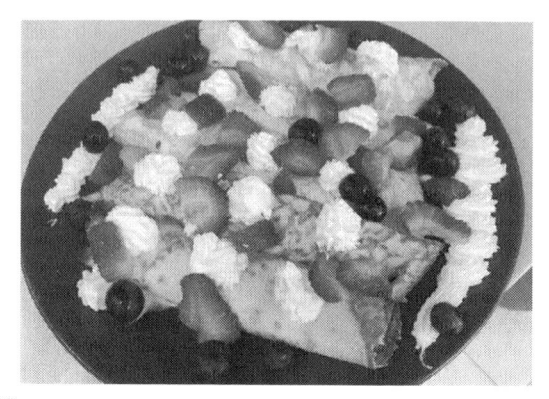

INGREDIENTS

- For the batter
- 2 - oz cream cheese full fat
- 2 - eggs
- Topping (optional)
- ½ - cup mixed berries
- 2 - tbsp heavy whipping cream
- Low Carb Crepes

INSTRUCTIONS

1. Warm up cream cheddar in a microwave so it motivates delicate and simple to blend
2. Add 2 eggs to cream cheddar (each one in turn) and blend well. Utilize a hand blender or a whisk. Add any flavors to the blend (discretionary)

3. Warm up a skillet, oil it marginally (I put some oil on an abundance and cleaned my skillet) and make your crepes.
4. Discretionary: You can make it sweet by including whipped cream, strawberries, berries, Greek yogurt, maple syrup and cinnamon. (Ensure it accommodates your macros.

Made in the USA
Middletown, DE
12 July 2019